Praise for *What Will Be*

"*What Will Be* brought me to tears. For anyone who has suffered from infertility and loss, this book shows you that you are not alone. It's a story of bravery, grit, and resilience, and of one woman's fight to never give up." —Reshma Saujani, founder of Girls Who Code

"Life can be unpredictable. It can be full of ups and downs. Sometimes, grief can suck everything out of you. In this beautiful, heartfelt memoir, Julie Pandya Patel reminds us that there's always hope. Infertility is a subject that simply is not discussed enough, as many suffer in silence. In this courageous story, the author puts everything out there, holding nothing back. Travel the emotional journey of a woman's quest to become a mother. Be ready to shed tears of sorrow, but more importantly, tears of joy. This story will stay with you." — Jalpa Williby, international award-winning and best-selling author of *My Perfect Imperfections*

WHAT WILL BE

*One Woman's Journey to Find
Inner Strength, Faith, and
Belief in the Impossible*

Julie Pandya Patel

ISBN 978-1-087-95426-4

Dedicated to

Samir, Sianna, and Kaia.

To infinity and beyond, I love you.

To all the women in the world who find themselves on a long journey to motherhood—your hopes, wishes, dreams, and faith are validated. There is no right or wrong path to motherhood. The path looks different for everyone.

CONTENTS

AUTHOR'S NOTE

I wrote this memoir to share the story of how my husband and I overcame the fertility challenges we faced when we decided to start a family. As a part of this journey, I researched many different treatments, supplements, and health practices recommended to boost fertility, which are mentioned throughout this book. I tried only the methods that I felt comfortable with. By no means am I suggesting that these same methods will necessarily work for others or lead to pregnancy. The decision to undergo fertility treatments is a personal choice that each woman must decide for herself. This book is not intended as a substitute for the medical advice of a physician. The reader should regularly consult a physician in matters relating to her health and particularly with respect to any symptoms that may require diagnosis or medical attention.

In addition, I have tried my best to recreate events, locales, and conversations based on my recollections of them. Some names and identifying details have been changed to protect the privacy of individuals.

WHAT WILL BE

PROLOGUE

I peed on the stick just like the box instructed. Then I placed it on the bathroom counter as the two-minute countdown began. I could have burned holes through that magic wand of a pregnancy test. That's how intently I was staring at the still-blank result window, waiting for a line to appear, for a sign, for something—anything—to end the agony of not knowing.

A pale blue line appeared, and then another intersected it like a cross. I couldn't believe it.

Are those two lines? Could it really be? Had years of trying, months of fertility treatments, countless supplements, yoga and acupuncture appointments, royal jelly and wretched-tasting wheatgrass finally resulted in the pregnancy Samir and I had hoped for so dearly?

I grabbed the test stick and looked at it again. I slid down to the floor in shock, my back to the wall. My hand was visibly shaking. *Two lines!*

I called Samir at work but got his voicemail. Now my entire body was shaking.

"Samir, it's me. Call me back, RIGHT AWAY."

I can't imagine what I must have sounded like. I called my sister next and could barely get the words out.

"Jalpa, I took a test...and I'm...I'm pregnant!"

*　　*　　*

When my husband, Samir, and I decided we wanted to get pregnant after a year of marriage, I was thirty-seven. I hadn't given a thought to the fact that we were in our late thirties and might face fertility challenges. I still felt like I was twenty-five.

I had always had a regular menstrual cycle, every twenty-eight days, like clockwork. I read up on tips for getting pregnant and talked to some friends who already had babies. I thought I had it covered. All we had to do was wait for Day 14 when I'd be ovulating, do the deed, and boom—I'd be pregnant, just like that.

Of course, I wasn't naive enough to think it would happen right away, but I thought in a few months, maybe five at most, we would be pregnant and on our way to starting our family. After all, my sister had three healthy kids and never had a problem conceiving, despite having her youngest child at thirty-eight. We had this in the bag.

But as the months wore on, and I celebrated my thirty-eighth birthday, I began to worry. I made an appointment to see the doctor.

My first meeting with Dr. Coffman, an experienced doctor at Northwestern Memorial Hospital with a stellar reputation, was one of the strangest meetings of my life. I had gone into our consultation thinking I'd come away reassured with some helpful advice. Instead, he launched into a full exploration of all the fertility treatments available to us. He showed me charts, went through diagrams, talked about the human body, described various treatment plans, circled and crossed off days on the calendar, highlighted hard-to-pronounce medical terms, and asked about meeting with Samir and getting him tested. Finally, he took my blood and sent me off. He told me they would call me with the results.

I walked out completely exhausted and confused with a manila folder filled with "options." Options for what exactly? How could he know that there was even a problem? Could I really be facing infertility?

Dr. Coffman had instructed me to go over everything with my husband. But I didn't know what to do or how to say it.

The reality that I might never ever become a mother hit me. And it hit me hard. How could I, Julie, the woman who has always enjoyed taking care of everyone around her, never be a mom?

Mothering others is a part of who I am. It is one of my most essential and deep-seated drives.

How many times had my friends told me, "You'll make a great mom one day." My friend Harleen had been calling me Mama Juls for years. I couldn't imagine a future version of my life that didn't include children of my own. Had I waited too long and missed my chance to start a family for good?

I tried my best to calm the panicked thoughts running through my head after that first meeting with Dr. Coffman and waited for the test results to come back. A few days later, the doctor's office called.

"All of your hormone levels from the blood work look normal. However, it looks like your AMH is low. It's less than .02."

"Oh, what should it be?" I asked.

"From about 1 to 3.5, but yours is so low, it's actually less than .02," the nurse explained from the other end of the phone. I wanted to scream, *No shit, I heard you!*

After we hung up, I spent hours googling "low AMH." Anti-Müllerian Hormone or AMH (an acronym that will forever haunt me) is a hormone given off by developing egg sacs that contain immature eggs. Measuring a woman's AMH levels is a way to gauge how many eggs she still has in reserve. My .02 reading meant I had very few viable eggs left. I could hear my heart beating through my chest when I finally deciphered this key fact. The odds were against me.

Screw the odds, I found myself thinking. *I'll prove them wrong.*

1

HOW I MET YOUR FATHER

The journey to becoming a mother doesn't just start when sperm meets egg. Of course, scientifically and biologically speaking, that is when the life of the embryo that later becomes your baby begins. But to start any story about motherhood there isn't really telling the whole story.

As much as I like to look back on the happy night my daughter Sianna was conceived or the day we finally brought her into this world, a healthy infant weighing 7 pounds, I know that to start this story there wouldn't be completely honest. It would mean omitting the entire time my husband and I spent trying to get pregnant: the frustrating doctor visits, the experimental treatments, the heartache of losing a baby to miscarriage, the fear of trying again. And before that, the years I spent working and living in the city as a single woman who was still searching for a partner to share my life with.

If you really want to know how I became a mother of two healthy girls, we have to start at the beginning when Sianna, my first daughter, was scarcely an idea in the back of my mind, much less a glint in my eye.

Like most women, I had imagined since I was a girl what it would be like to get married: the wedding, the beautiful sarees I'd get to wear, and the man who would sweep me off my feet. But it wasn't something I fixated on or tried to schedule into my life by a certain age. I'd had several long-term boyfriends throughout college and my twenties. I figured I'd meet my true love and get married as a matter of course, when the time was right.

Then I turned thirty—that age when women the world over suddenly register their biological clocks ticking away at an accelerated clip. Exiting my twenties was like saying goodbye to simpler times when life revolved around career and friends; dating was not something I had to take too seriously. Things were different in my thirties. I wanted more than just a spark of chemistry or attraction. I was looking for a partner, and not just any partner, but the right one.

The pressure mounted as I watched many of my close friends meet and marry their life partners and then start families of their own.

My sister, Jalpa, who is eight years older, had married when she was twenty-eight and already had three kids. I was the baby of the family, and my parents were beginning to get nervous. I was officially AMA, as many people in our Indian community liked to say: Advanced Marital Age. Mom, accordingly, reached out to every auntie and uncle in the Chicago metropolitan area and even our relatives in India to look for a suitable match.

"What about so-and-so, who is a family friend of Gautam Uncle? Couldn't you at least meet him for a coffee?" my mom would suggest not-so-subtly over the phone.

I tried my best to shrug off my parents' well-meaning suggestions. Even friends had begun to offer their match-making skills to me.

Dating in my thirties was no cakewalk. I was on as many dating sites as I had the time to manage. But whether I was on Match or Shaadi, a dating service that pitches itself as "the No.1 Matchmaking service for Desi Singles" in the US, the results were always the same. I kept meeting guys who, after a few dates, I realized were just not right for me. Some of them were barely able to commit to a dinner date, much less a serious relationship with marriage potential further down the line.

It was depressing. My friends told me to hang in there, that it was a numbers game. By the time I turned thirty-four, nearly all my close friends were married or engaged to be married. My social calendar revolved around engagement parties and extravagant weddings, followed by baby showers and children's birthday parties.

That summer, my friends Sapna and Nirav invited me to their son Kavin's first birthday. Sapna and her husband were throwing a big party to celebrate the milestone. Single and childless, I dreaded driving out to their flawless home in the suburbs. But Sapna had always been a good friend to me, so I knew it was important that I showed up to celebrate this moment in her son's life.

I listened to music on the drive out to the suburbs, but it was mostly drowned out by the subconscious voice in the back of my head that kept asking, Would I ever throw a first birthday party for my baby someday?

Sapna and Nirav's house was packed when I arrived. There must have been at least a hundred people there, including a number of babies and toddlers, and the house was decorated with balloons and streamers. I made a deal with myself that I'd eat some food and stay just long enough to watch them blow out the candles and serve cake. Then I'd peace out and head to my parents' house for the weekend for some rest and relaxation.

I made my way to the backyard where the BBQ was set up and people were generally chatting and hanging out. As I was loading up my plate at the buffet table, preparing to eat my feelings, I felt a light tap on my shoulder.

"Hey, Julie? Is that you?"

I turned and saw two familiar faces looking back at me. It was Barry and Samir, old friends who went way back.

"Oh, hey, Samir! Barry! I haven't seen you guys in forever."

I was relieved to see I wasn't the only one who had come to the party without a date or spouse. The guys grabbed some food from the buffet and then we sat down at one of the tables outside. It turned out we all lived in the city. Barry was married, but as far as I could gather, Samir was still single, and the guys had carpooled out to Sapna and Nirav's house. In fact, Samir's apartment was only a few miles from mine.

"You mean I could have caught a ride with you guys?" I complained jokingly. "Damn. I guess there's always Kavin's next birthday, right?"

I hadn't seen Samir in years, maybe not since right after I graduated from college. I'd first met him and his group of guy friends as a sixteen year old. Me and my two best friends, who both happened to be named Reshma, had begged one of the Reshma's older sisters,

Keshma, to let us tag along with her one Saturday night. We were sheltered kids from the suburbs and, like teenage girls everywhere, desperate to get out and hang with the cool kids.

Every weekend we had the chance, we'd go to parties with Keshma. Samir and the rest of the guys had always seemed tough and street wise. They were older and had grown up in Chicago—the city, not the suburbs of Schaumburg, Illinois. They were definitely cool and had an edge to them.

I was pleasantly surprised to run into Samir, especially since I had forgotten he was such a music junkie like me. He said he still went to a lot of concerts and was always looking for opportunities to see musical acts live, so we agreed to keep in touch through Facebook. It hadn't escaped my notice that Samir had cleaned up since college—he looked different, more mature.

What about Samir? I found myself thinking after I left the party and drove over to my parents' place. He was chill, had a good job, loved music. And I had known him for years. *Maybe*, I thought and filed the idea away.

*   *   *

A month or so later, on a quiet night at home alone, I sent Samir a message on Facebook.

> Hey Samir, how's it going? Been to any fun
> concerts lately?

That's how it started. For the next few months, we continued to chat about the bands we'd seen or the new music we were listening to, but we still hadn't made any plans to meet in person. As the fall approached, the days filled up with holiday plans and family obligations and our messages slowed to a drip.

I was home on a Friday night after a long week at work, watching TV, when my phone pinged on the coffee table. It was a message from Samir.

> Hey, what are you up to? Any chance you want to go
> see The Fray tonight?

I did a double take when I first read the message. Did he know The Fray was my favorite band? I hadn't even known they were in town. Of course I wanted to see them! I responded immediately and without hesitation.

> Yes!! I love The Fray!

> Awesome. Send me your number.

I messaged him my number and he called me right away. The show, which was part of The Fray's Miracle Near State Street tour, was set to start at 9:30 p.m. at the Auditorium Theatre. It was already 8 p.m., but the theater was only a few blocks away from my apartment. He didn't have tickets but felt sure we could get some.

"People are always scalping tickets on the street," Samir said. Famous last words.

An hour later, as I walked up to the theatre, I could see Samir standing out front in a grey trench coat. *Wow*, I thought, *he looks good*. He seemed a bit frustrated, though. We hugged and said hello, before he dropped the news.

"You're gonna kill me," he started, "I can't get tickets. I tried, but the guy at the box office won't sell me any. I don't know what to do."

My heart sunk for a moment. Here we were, finally, hanging out in person on a maybe-date and now we couldn't actually get into the show. And it wasn't just any show. It was the sold-out performance of my favorite band in the world, and they were in Chicago for one night only. We had to find a way in.

"Okay, let me try," I said, resolving not to come back empty-handed. I went in and headed straight for the ticket booth. But the man's response was the same.

"You really don't have any tickets left? I'm willing to pay whatever they cost," I pleaded.

"I'm sorry, honey," the clerk answered, "Believe me, if I had any tickets left, I'd gladly sell them to you."

I walked back outside where Samir was waiting. I didn't have to say anything because the disappointment was written all over my face.

"Well, at least we tried," Samir offered.

Just then, a blonde woman and her husband exited the theater doors we were standing next to. She said something to her husband, then turned and looked at us.

"Do you guys need tickets?" she asked.

It was as if this woman had appeared out of nowhere like a guardian angel who had been sent to help us in our hour of need. My mouth dropped. All I could do was stare at the crisp white tickets she was holding out in her hand.

"We have to go. We have an emergency," she tried again.

"Yes, we'll take them!" Samir replied since I was too tongue-tied to get a word out. "Can we pay you for them?"

"No, no. Just go and enjoy the show," the woman reassured us with a smile. Then she and her husband ran down the block to hail a taxi and disappeared into the night.

"Oh my god! Can you believe this?" I practically shouted, I was so giddy with excitement.

"No. It's a miracle!" Samir said, shaking his head with incredulity. We hugged and jumped up and down to celebrate. It was 9:25 pm by this point, so we hurried into the theater to take our seats.

We handed the usher our tickets and she led us to our seats in the second row, center stage. Samir and I looked at each other. There were no words that could describe the shock and awe we were both experiencing. Ten minutes before, we had been stuck outside without a chance of getting into the show. And now, we were sitting two rows from the stage.

The Fray rocked the stage that night, and we had an incredible time, dancing and singing along to the songs. It was an epic night to remember. Years later, we would often look back on it and say, "Thank God for the Miracle Near State Street."

2

FIRST COMES LOVE, THEN COMES MARRIAGE

After Samir and I had experienced our own little miracle that December night at The Fray concert, we began spending a lot of time together. Samir wasn't like the other guys I had dated. One of the things that made him so different, in an era of texting, was that when we couldn't hang out in person, he would call me instead. We often spent hours on the phone in deep conversation.

The truth is I was smitten—and I trusted Samir because I'd known him since I was a teenager. Pretty soon, as things progressed into the new year, we decided it was time to share the news of us "going steady" with our mutual friends.

One day after I had just seen Samir, I met up with one of my best friends, Jankhana. She noticed something was different almost immediately.

"What's gotten into you? You look so happy."

I was grinning from ear to ear and hadn't even realized it. I told her that I'd met someone and when I said who it was, she couldn't believe it.

"Samir Patel? No, you're joking. You've known him since you were a kid. And now, after all these years . . . ?"

"I know," I admitted, "It's crazy. But he's such a great guy."

Talk of our courtship began to spread little by little. A few weekends later, Samir had plans to go watch Sunday football with friends. I decided to tag along, so when his friend Shailes came to pick us up and saw me, he had to do a double take.

"Hey, Julie. I didn't know you were coming. Wait a sec, are you guys . . . dating?"

Samir and I both nodded in response, giddy smiles plastered on our faces.

Though surprised at first by our unforeseen pairing, everyone was overwhelmingly happy for us, especially our parents. Samir is three years older than me, so his parents had been wondering whether he would ever settle down as well.

2010 was the year our relationship blossomed. I was certain about Samir—that he was the right person for me, that I wanted to spend the rest of my life with him—in a way that I had never been in any other relationship.

From the very beginning, I had envisioned what our life together might look like. So by early 2011, I was ready for Samir to pop the question. But I didn't know if he was.

A week before Valentine's Day that year, I brought up the subject. I asked him where our relationship was headed and said I was ready for the next step. I was caught completely off guard by his answer: Samir wasn't ready. We were out of sync, on separate pages, different wavelengths.

I tried not to panic, but I was worried. I didn't want to push the issue any further, though, so I accepted his answer at face value and suggested maybe we could revisit the idea in a few months. In reality, I was crushed. Samir was the one—but what if he didn't feel the same way?

The next weekend Samir had planned a business trip to Los Angeles. He wouldn't be back in time for Valentine's Day, so we agreed we'd celebrate when he got back to Chicago. On Thursday, the night before he was to leave, I went over to his apartment to hang out while he packed. He told me there was something in the kitchen for me, so I walked into the next room to take a look. There, sitting on the table, was a card addressed to me. It read:

> Happy Valentine's Weekend! Pack your bags because you're getting on a plane tomorrow headed for LA.

My heart melted. Samir was still the man I had fallen in love with, spontaneous and fun-loving. He had even cleared the day off from work with my boss. We flew out to LA together the next day and had an amazing weekend. Who doesn't love seventy-degree sunshine in the middle of winter?

On Sunday morning I opened my eyes groggily to see Samir kneeling next to my bedside, holding a large box.

"What's this?" I managed, after wiping the sleep from my eyes and waking up enough to realize this was not a dream.

"Open it," Samir said with a mischievous grin.

I followed his instructions and opened the box to reveal a large, black leather purse. It was sleek and stylish, but it seemed like a strange gift to wake somebody up for. I looked back at Samir, and he cocked his head to one side.

"Look inside," he said.

"Okay . . . ," I responded, even more puzzled.

I reached my hand inside the black bag and pulled out a smaller, red leather purse. Sensing that there was something else a foot here, I continued to unzip the red purse—and that's when my heart stopped. Inside was a box. Not just any kind of box, but a jewelry box, the kind you always see the moment before someone is about to propose.

Before I could even utter a word, Samir slid the box into his hands.

"Julie Pandya, will you make me the happiest man in the world—will you marry me?"

As he said those fateful words, he opened the box to reveal a stunning ring. I was absolutely speechless. I nodded emphatically as tears streamed down my face and then finally squeaked out, "Yes! The answer is yes."

I grabbed Samir by the shoulders and made him stand up so that we could hug. The surprises didn't end there, however. Since our relationship had begun with music and that special concert with The Fray, he wanted to commemorate our engagement with another musical milestone. This time it was the Grammys! The annual music award show with all the biggest names from the music industry. I couldn't believe it! I don't know how Samir pulled it off, but he had worked the phones for months until he somehow had secured tickets for the two of us.

The show was that very night, so we had little time to spare. We sprinted off to Bloomingdales to get outfitted in Grammy-ready attire: Samir in a slick suit and me in a glittery, sequined outfit. We had the time of our lives, rocking out in the crowd as Rihanna strutted across the stage for the TV cameras. I remember catching the sparkle from the ring now perched on my left hand and then staring at it in disbelief. I couldn't believe it—we were finally getting married.

*　　　*　　　*

When we got back to Chicago, there was no shortage of hugs and laughs from family and friends. Their joy for us was contagious. I launched straight into planning the wedding. Jankhana gave me some advice when she heard of our engagement: "Don't wait to get married. It will only prolong everything else down the line." Little did I know then how true her words would ring later.

Things fell into place fairly quickly. We found a venue that could accommodate a traditional Indian wedding, which usually consists of three days of ceremonies and activities, and were lucky enough to secure Labor Day weekend for the festivities. We settled on the date of September 4, 2011. It felt right since our first date had been December 4, 2009.

Seven months later, Samir and I were sitting in the ballroom of the Renaissance Hotel and surveying the room filled with more than

400 friends and family as husband and wife. Those three days were filled with colorful outfits, delicious food, a lot of love, and a beautiful wedding followed by dancing through the night. It was one of the happiest times of my life.

The morning after the wedding ended, our parents and wedding party gave us an enthusiastic sendoff as we hopped into a car headed for the airport. We would spend our three-week honeymoon in Australia and Bora Bora.

*　　*　　*

Our honeymoon consisted of three glorious weeks of sunshine, excursions into the Australian outback, and romantic dinners with breathtaking views of the Pacific Ocean. I came back with a tan and that special post-honeymoon glow. Samir and I were so happy together. It all felt like a fairy tale.

Now that we were husband and wife, Samir moved into my apartment, and we began consolidating our things into one home. Colleagues at work and acquaintances continued to wish us congratulations for achieving one of life's biggest milestones. Of course, the first question people ask newlyweds, predictably, is, "So, when are you going to start popping out kids?"

Samir and I knew we wanted to start a family, but at the same time, I hadn't caught the motherhood bug and didn't yet feel a sense of urgency around getting pregnant. We stopped using protection once we were married and figured things would take their natural course. Sooner or later, I assumed, I'd get pregnant. But it wasn't something I was going to worry about. We'd simply cross that bridge when we got there.

The end of 2011 turned into 2012 and our first year of marriage flew by with it. We celebrated our first wedding anniversary in September 2012. In all that time there hadn't been any signs of pregnancy, not even a false alarm like a late or missed period. Still, I hadn't been too concerned about it.

Then in December, I went with a bunch of girlfriends on a trip to the Kohler Waters Spa, a retreat in Wisconsin, to celebrate our friend Sapna's birthday. One afternoon, a few of us went to get massages. As the masseuses worked their magic, Sweety, a mutual friend, and I chatted casually. I told her about Samir and how we were enjoying our first year of marriage. She told me about her work as a nurse.

"Do you want to have kids?" she asked matter-of-factly.

It had been a while since anyone had posed that question to me and not in a joking way, the way people do when you're fresh off your honeymoon.

"Yes, we do want children. We've been trying to let things take their natural course, but so far we haven't gotten pregnant." It was only when I said these words aloud, in the company of other people, that I began to worry that maybe something was wrong. Sweety made me really think. My friend Jankhana's words came back to me. "Don't wait," she had said. And now it had been more than a year since we stopped using protection.

"I worked with an awesome fertility doctor at Northwestern Memorial Hospital," Sweety suggested. "I'd be happy to refer you to him. His name is Dr. Coffman."

"Thanks. I really appreciate the offer and will think about it," I said.

Think about it I did—that's when the fear started to wiggle its way into my psyche. *Why haven't we gotten pregnant in nearly fifteen months of trying without birth control? What if something is wrong? What if we can't get pregnant at all?*

3

THE DOCTOR WILL SEE YOU NOW

Despite the misgivings my conversation in the massage room stoked at the Kohler Waters Spa, life went on as normal. Christmas and New Year's passed quickly into the arrival of January and February, and with those first months of the year, came the deep chill of winter in Chicago. By March, Samir and I and everyone else we knew were predictably worn out by the below-freezing temperatures.

My birthday on March 13—I was turning thirty-eight this year —was just around the corner and offered a welcome distraction to break up the winter doldrums. Samir planned a dinner at a Mediterranean place called Kan Zaman and invited a group of my closest girlfriends and their significant others. The restaurant was lavishly decorated with beaded lampshades and artwork on the walls;

the banquette along the far wall was lined with round brass tables; handwoven rugs and furs were draped over the seats; and the low lighting gave the room an intimate feel.

The restaurant even had a belly dancer to entertain guests. She slowly shimmied her way around the table, before stopping at my chair where she beckoned me to join her. Against my better judgment, I got up and tried to copy her fluid movements as our impromptu dance lesson ensued. My friends cheered me on in between bouts of laughter, though it was clear belly dancing was not my forte.

At one point during the night, I looked around the dinner table and surveyed my closest friends joined in lively conversation as they ate from hearty entrées and platters of salad, hummus, and kabob. My heart swelled with gratitude and happiness at the scene before my eyes. We had all grown so much over the course of our friendship, becoming successful professionals, finding life partners. I felt blessed to be a part of this loving group of people and for the wonderful birthday dinner Samir had planned. We had so much to be thankful for and indeed we were.

We capped the night off by moving to a nearby lounge so that we could continue to hang out and chat. The entire evening had been a wonderful way to celebrate another year. And yet, I was becoming more and more conscious of something I had wanted and put off for a long time now: motherhood.

I had met and married my partner in life. We both had stable, well-paying jobs, a comfortable home, close friends, and an extended family who were always there to support us. The moment was finally right to start a family. So what was holding us back?

Perhaps it was time to put in a more concerted effort. I thought it would only be right to start by seeing a doctor who could dispense some expert advice and point us in the right direction. Samir agreed when I mentioned the idea to him. Why not get checked out first to make sure everything was okay? Then we could focus more intentionally on making a baby.

Not wanting to stir up talk or any unwanted attention—deciding to start a family and trying to get pregnant is a deeply personal decision—I didn't reach out to Sweety to get the doctor's referral. I remembered enough of the details from our conversation that I was able to do a simple Google search. Dr. Coffman popped right up; his reputation, it seemed, preceded him. I called up the number at Northwestern Memorial Hospital and made an appointment for a few weeks later. And that was that, so I thought.

*   *   *

On the morning of my appointment, I got dressed for work, ate a quick breakfast, kissed Samir goodbye, and then walked to the hospital, which was only a few blocks away from our apartment. The plan was to pop in for an early appointment and then arrive at work a little after my normal start time.

When I stepped into the fertility department's waiting room, I immediately noticed how bright and clean it was. The magazines were neatly stacked on various coffee tables; the water cooler was fully stocked with paper cups; the receptionists were friendly and welcoming. I filled out a few necessary forms and then sat down to wait for my name to be called.

It was still early, but the office was already buzzing with activity. People were coming in and out. Some women had arrived alone, while others sat waiting with their partners. It occurred to me that we were all there for the same reason, but our common cause didn't seem to make the fact of being there—waiting to see a fertility doctor—any easier. No one made eye contact with me as I scanned the room. Everyone seemed to be keeping themselves occupied by flipping through magazines or browsing their phones. Perhaps we were all nervous and maybe even a bit embarrassed about our own situations. Infertility was a taboo subject, something we had been socialized not to talk about in polite conversation. So many of us felt shame because of it, blaming ourselves for something that was out of our control.

"Julie Patel?" one of the nurses called out, clipboard in hand. I stood up and followed the nurse through a door and down a hallway until we arrived at Dr. Coffman's office. It was a small room with a large wooden desk. The doctor was sitting behind it, but as soon as I entered, he stood up to greet me and shake my hand.

As I sat down, I felt a few beads of perspiration begin to collect on my palms. Sitting in his office suddenly made everything feel real.

"So, Mrs. Patel, tell me about yourself," Dr. Coffman said with genuine interest in a vaguely European accent.

Though he was nearing retirement, it was clear that Dr. Coffman still took joy in getting to know new patients. I was also relieved to start our appointment with something innocuous. I happily told him how Samir and I had known each other since our teenage years and only begun seeing each other romantically when we reconnected in our thirties; that we both grew up in Indian households with the same values; that Samir worked in finance, while I had transitioned to the nonprofit world and then back to finance; that we'd been married for more than a year and half and had stopped using protection, but so far nothing had happened; that we both felt ourselves getting older and wanted to start a family before time ran out.

He nodded and smiled as I told him our story. When I finished, he told me a little about himself: Dr. Coffman had been treating patients struggling with infertility for many years and had delivered thousands of healthy babies over his long tenure.

"Don't you worry, Mrs. Patel. My specialty is to help people make babies," he reassured me. I appreciated his lighthearted sense of humor, which eased some of my own nervousness.

I also learned that Dr. Coffman was well-traveled and had taken a special interest in Indian culture and food. He told me about his trip to India and all the amazing things he had eaten there. Sitting in his office and chatting in this way was like getting lunch with an old friend —natural and unhurried.

Eventually, though, we did have to get to the reason I'd showed up at his office in the first place. Dr. Coffman suggested we start with an overview of human biology and how the female body works. He brought out various charts and graphs as he explained the ins and outs of egg development, ovulation, and menstruation—topics I'd thought I understood because I was born a woman, but as it turned out, there was much more to it than what I'd studied in high school biology.

He proceeded to explain the different things that often go wrong when a couple tries to conceive. In order to figure out what was going on in our situation, he would need to take blood samples from me and Samir and conduct several other tests.

Although Dr. Coffman had gone through everything in the most gentle and thoughtful way, it was an overwhelming amount of information to take in. My head was still spinning when he jumped ahead to potential treatments, which, of course, would be determined by what our test results showed. *But we don't even know if there's really a problem*, I thought as I felt my heart flutter. *Oh my god, there might be a problem.*

"Let's get your blood drawn today and set up an appointment for Samir to come in as well, and then we'll take it from there," Dr. Coffman said. "How does that sound? Julie—does that sound OK?"

The thought that we might not be able to get pregnant had just hit me and sent me into a silent panic. I looked up and saw Dr. Coffman still waiting for my answer.

"Yes, that sounds great. Thank you so much, Doctor," I finally managed.

The rest of that day was a blur. Dr. Coffman sent me home with a packet of papers explaining everything we had gone over. I remembered returning to work, but honestly, I doubt I got much of anything done that day. I spent a good portion of it googling infertility problems and their treatments and success rates.

At home that evening, I pulled out the stack of papers and told Samir how the appointment had gone, expressing my surprise at how much more serious things might be. In his characteristic calm, Samir said simply, "We have to do what we have to do."

*　　*　　*

We made an appointment for me and Samir to go into see Dr. Coffman together the next week. A few days beforehand, I received a call from one of the nurses about my blood test results.

"All of your hormone levels from the blood work look normal," she said, at which I was ready to heave a sigh of relief. I could feel a "but" coming, though. It was something in the tone of her voice. "However, it looks like your AMH is low. It's less than .02," she concluded.

I had no idea what that meant or whether I should be concerned. So I asked what my "AMH" should be.

"From about 1 to 3.5, but yours is so low it's actually less than .02," she clarified as if it were the most obvious thing in the world. My eyes widened and every follicle in my body wanted to rear up and scream. I was at work receiving this news on my cell phone at my desk, so screaming was out of the question. Instead, my emotions raged in silence. I thanked the nurse and hung up. After which, I immediately opened a new Google browser window and spiraled ever deeper into the inter webs on infertility.

AMH stood for Anti-Müllerian Hormone, I soon learned. It's a hormone that is present in women when they have healthy developing eggs in their ovaries. The fact that I had so little of it suggested a low number of eggs, or at least a very low number of viable ones. No eggs, no baby.

That one phone call whipped me up into a frenzy of worry and regret. What if it was too late for us to get pregnant? Why hadn't we tried sooner?

Even though I didn't fully understand the "low AMH" result I'd been given, I knew now for sure why we hadn't gotten pregnant on our own. There was a problem. For the first time in my life, I realized that becoming a mother was not a given, not something I could take for granted, and very likely a thing I would have to fight hard for if I truly wanted it.

Several days after my blood results had rocked our world, Samir and I went into the doctor's office for our follow-up appointment. Samir was sent off to another room so that he could give a semen sample (I'm sure this was something he'd never imagined he'd have to do). Afterward, we sat down in Dr. Coffman's office and went over my results together.

Dr. Coffman discussed what low AMH meant for us, but didn't linger on the number. He also explained that I had fibroids, but said they shouldn't affect our chances at pregnancy. Overall, I had a healthy uterus and that was good news. His MO was to focus on the good. From his point of view, it wasn't about "if" we would get pregnant, but rather a matter of "when."

Although we didn't yet have the results from Samir's tests, Dr. Coffman walked us through our next options and put together a game plan. I felt better knowing that there was a way forward with several different treatments we could try. He reassured us that we'd done the right thing. We had come in early enough to diagnose the situation and now we could proactively create the best conditions for a potential future pregnancy.

"We'll take things one step at a time," Dr. Coffman said with confidence. Helping people bring life into the world was his passion and his expertise. His positivity was uplifting, and given his successful track record, we had every reason to believe, as he did, that we would one day be parents. They say you have to dream it to believe it.

4
DAY 3

E ven though the odds of getting pregnant were slim, I tried to stay positive and look for the silver lining. I was thankful, at least, that I could count on my regular menstrual cycle. After spending hours reading dozens of articles on Google, I knew that many women didn't even have that to rely on, making the process of timing fertility treatments even more daunting.

Dr. Coffman recommended a regimen of Clomid, a fertility drug that helps stimulate egg follicles by increasing the amount of hormones that support the growth and release of mature eggs, in turn inducing ovulation. I was to take Clomid in combination with intrauterine insemination (IUI) over the course of three months. The IUI would essentially inject my husband's sperm into my uterus to help the sperm get into the fallopian tube quicker and fertilize my eggs. We decided to start immediately once my next cycle began. On Day 3 of my menstrual cycle, I went in to the doctor's office to get my blood drawn as instructed.

This was May of 2013. At the time, I was handling residential mortgage transactions at a top firm in Corporate America, but I still felt I had to hide my infertility issues. I didn't want to tell anyone what Samir and I were going through. I had to be at work at 8:30 a.m. every day, which meant arriving at the doctor's at 7 a.m. to get my blood drawn so that I could make it to work on time. Then, I waited until the afternoon to receive a call from the doctor's office. They told me all my hormone levels were where they should be at that point in my cycle and that it would be okay to move forward with the Clomid and IUI course of action. They had sent the prescription for Clomid to my pharmacy, and I was instructed to take one pill daily starting on Day 5 through Day 9 of my cycle. On Day 9, I would go in for an ultrasound to see how my eggs were developing. I was supposed to go in every other day until the eggs reached 14 mm-16 mm, at which point they would give me an Ovidrel shot to help trigger ovulation. One day after the shot, we would come in for the IUI.

When you experience difficult seasons in life and feel you have no control over the way you want things to go, you start to appreciate the small things. I didn't relish the routine fertility treatments—no one does—but I was comforted by the fact that my doctor was genuinely concerned about my case and I was being cared for at one of the top hospitals in the country. The clinic was close enough to my home that I could walk there, and the spring weather was getting nicer by the day.

Once Samir's tests came back, we got the official OK to move forward with the IUI treatment plan, and I began taking the Clomid pills. I took them every day of my cycle until Day 9, then I went in for ultrasounds starting on Day 10 to see what the eggs in my fallopian tubes were measuring at. I appreciated the ultrasound machines at this clinic because they had a screen where I could view what the ultrasound was seeing in real time. Whenever the doctor found any egg activity in my fallopian tubes, I smiled excitedly at the screen. This gave me something tangible to have faith in. I went in every other day until Day 14. Once the doctor found an egg that measured 16 mm, he called us in for an Ovidrel shot the next day, and an IUI the day after that. We went in with high hopes and high spirits for our first IUI that May. Always optimistic, I was certain it would work.

After the procedure, the doctors advised staying in the hospital bed for about twenty minutes to avoid disrupting the magic going on inside my body and to give my husband's swimmers the best chance of making it to the mothership: my growing egg.

I remember this first time so vividly. Samir and I were so excited and happy. We recognized how lucky we were to have access to this treatment option. We felt like we were taking control of our destiny—and it made us giddy. To celebrate the moment, my husband played a song from Depeche Mode on his phone, his all-time favorite band, and placed it right on my uterus. We just knew we were going to have our Depeche Mode baby. Man, were we naive.

Once the IUI is administered, you are required to wait two weeks (any woman who is trying to get pregnant is aware of this dreaded but hopeful two-week waiting period better known as the "2 week wait" or 2WW) and hope your period doesn't come. After my first IUI, I made the decision to stop drinking any alcohol and caffeine during the two-week waiting period. For me, it was giving up something minor for something much bigger. I prayed every day. I went into work but my mind wasn't really there.

Every chance I got, me and my new best friend—Google—sat side by side. I read everything I could about the 2WW. For example, I read about the various things you can do to increase your chances of pregnancy, including herbal medicine, fertility yoga, acupuncture, CoQ10, wheatgrass, and so many more supplements. Whenever these techniques confused me or made me feel overwhelmed by all the things I suddenly learned I should be doing, I read success stories from other women with low AMH levels in fertility message boards. Their stories gave me so much hope and helped me believe it was possible for me too. I'll never forget the many mothers who were brave enough to pour their hearts out and talk about their fertility journeys to other strangers on the internet—just to help someone else who was now in the same position they had once been in. I vowed silently that after I gave birth to a healthy baby, I would share my story to help out anyone I could.

Embarking on this journey of getting pregnant and starting a family, with the help of doctors, nurses, and modern science, was an intensely private decision for us. I hadn't told any of my friends and certainly none of my professional colleagues. My parents and in-laws had been pestering Samir and me since the day after our wedding about giving them grandchildren. My mom knew that we were trying, but I resisted the urge to tell her about the program of fertility treatments. It would be too hard to explain the ins and outs of Clomid and IUIs to an Indian mother. My sister was the only person I confided in since she had been like a second mom to me my whole life. None of our other relatives knew. There is such a stigma that comes with infertility, yet in reality, women all over the world suffer from these issues regularly.

By Day 9 of our first fertility treatment, I started symptom checking. I had never been pregnant before, so I was hyper-sensitive to every little twinge, ache, or feeling that seemed out of the ordinary. I was sure I was pregnant and couldn't wait to take the pregnancy test. I waited until Day 11 to test. I had read that sometimes you could test positive as early as Day 9 and thought that could be me! On Day 11, the test returned negative. I tested again the next day—negative. I continued to check for any symptoms. I was convinced I was pregnant because I felt different. I was bloated and hungrier than usual, already craving specific foods. Day 13—negative again. But I'm cramping, I thought. Isn't that a definite sign of early pregnancy? Day 14— negative. That's okay, I thought, I'll get my positive tomorrow.

At 2 p.m. at work the next day, I got my period. I walked back to my desk from the bathroom with an unusual sense of calmness, considering how fixated I had been on my pregnancy "symptoms" all week. I felt nothing. Maybe I went numb and didn't want to think about the fact that we would have to repeat these daunting steps again next month. All I could think was, *It will happen next time.* My brain knew there could only be one outcome—the one I was so desperately wishing and yearning for—so it protected me and let me continue believing it was going to happen. I spent the rest of the day eerily composed.

I'm okay, I kept thinking to myself. *We have next month.* But I dreaded telling Samir. The guilt of feeling like it was my fault—my body's fault—that we couldn't get pregnant was beginning to set in. I felt his frustration and my own at all the appointments, the doctor consultations, the tests, and most of all, the agonizing uncertainty of every day that passed. It felt so unfair, but I told myself that God challenges you for a reason. *I have to stay positive. I can handle this.*

I called my doctor's office to tell them I got my period. Since I had begun a new menstrual cycle, they told me to come in for lab work and that we would start the process again. On Day 3, I went into the doctor's at 7 a.m. *Here we go.*

That next month during our 2WW, Samir and I decided to go out with some friends over the weekend. It was June, the best time of the year to be in Chicago, and summertime was just beginning to bloom. At this point, people had been holed up inside, away from the harsh winter weather, for months. Lounging at the packed rooftop bar at the Wit Hotel downtown, soaking up the sunshine, it felt as though the city was buzzing—as if people had never seen the sun before.

It was great to be out, enjoying the weather and our friends' company, but if I were honest with myself, I didn't really want to be there. The pressures of following and keeping up with all the fertility procedures, check-ups, and prescriptions, as well as dealing emotionally with our disappointing results thus far, had begun to weigh on me and Samir. Our relationship was unusually tense. We argued more often. Both of us wanted to bring a baby into the world and start the next chapter of our life together, but the stress was beginning to push us apart. I knew that going out for the day with friends, as frivolous as that sounds, was something Samir needed. He needed to feel the normalcy of our former lives, even if only for a brief moment.

So I put on makeup and dragged myself out into the sunlight that Saturday afternoon, but I continued to stick with the vow I had made to myself when we started fertility treatments: no drinks during the 2WW period. Luckily, Shaila, one of my good friends, was there and she was seven months pregnant, so we kept each other company while our husbands enjoyed cocktails. What I had failed to anticipate were the watchful eyes. A few hours into this impromptu rooftop party, I noticed that people were looking at me differently. They thought I was pregnant just because I didn't have a drink in my hand.

I was dressed fashionably in an off-the-shoulder black top tucked into shorts and black high heels that strapped around my ankle. I didn't think I looked pregnant, even though I hoped that I was. I was pretty sure I looked exactly like I did the last time they saw me a month prior. I had never even considered the idea that friends might be on the lookout to see whether Samir and I were trying to start a family. All I could do was look down or glance away as their gazes followed me.

As the day went on and people became tipsier, I heard someone say, "Oh, for sure she's pregnant." My heart sank. Though the words themselves carried no bad intentions, they hit me like a ton of bricks. If only they knew how bad I wished those words were true.

That very morning, I had my second IUI procedure. If only they knew about the anxiety I went through the night before, about the hole in the pit of my stomach that had been filling with dread and worry since I woke up, about the waves of nervousness that washed over me as I laid on the hospital bed and waited several hours for the insemination procedure. If only they knew how emotionally and physically drained my husband and I were, how I didn't even want to join them at brunch and would have rather curled up in the bed after my procedure. If only they knew.

So I smiled and continued to sip my club soda. We had been so carefree and open before, so involved in enjoying our life together. We had no restrictions—we did whatever we wanted, whenever we wanted, and now things were changing rapidly. Being so focused on our fertility plan registered a fundamental shift in my mind; I couldn't be my carefree self anymore. I knew at that point that our life together would never be the same. I would never be the same. When we got home that night, neither of us said a word about brunch. We both went straight to bed. *Wow, that was exhausting*, was all I could think.

During the day, I found myself making doctors' appointments, calling pharmacies for our fertility prescriptions, and often being put on hold for almost half an hour at work while my boss angrily glared at me. I practically snarled whenever a colleague asked if I wanted a cup of coffee or tea (I'd been off caffeine for more than a month). One thing we did have on our side was we were fortunate enough to have health insurance that covered a lot of the costs associated with the meds and procedures so far. I couldn't imagine what it would have been like with the added stress of bearing the financial burden of fertility treatments on our own, a challenge that many families who don't have insurance coverage face daily.

A few nights later, Samir said to me, "Hey J, it's okay if we don't have a baby. We have each other. We can enjoy life, travel, and be completely happy." He realized the desire to get pregnant had taken over our life. And he was absolutely right. However, this sent me into a tailspin. I remembered a time before we got married—Samir once told me that he could imagine the children we would have together. Even though he didn't express it, I knew how important it was for him to grow our family. I was determined to stay focused, even if it meant losing ourselves for a little bit to make this wish become a reality for both of us. I had one response to his statement: "No way, we are having a baby."

Then, the next IUI failed.

I fell asleep that night dreading the next month of fertility treatments that awaited us. But as I slumbered, a reassuring vision came to me. I imagined her, my daughter, in my dreams. Even now, I can still see her tiny round face wrapped up in a pink blanket, every detail in its place.

In my dream, her daddy played airplane with her. He was full of joy, laughing in the delivery room. He took her in his arms and zoomed her playfully through the air. I laughed while the nurses scolded him, reminding him that she was just a newborn.

"This is my daughter," he said proudly.

The dream was so vivid, I had no doubt that it would come to fruition. This I knew: that was my daughter in my dreams, and one day, she would be in my arms.

5
FINDING MY TRIBE

Although Samir and I were crestfallen after the second IUI failed, and the regimen of fertility treatments was both physically and emotionally draining, I wasn't ready to give up. I was convinced deep down in the core of my being that we were going to get pregnant. We just hadn't exhausted every avenue yet.

So I began to focus more on holistic approaches. I scoured the internet for stories of women with low AMH who successfully became pregnant, and as a result I became well-versed in seemingly every trick in the book for boosting your chances of conceiving. I had a long list of new age therapies like acupuncture, royal jelly, fertility yoga, and wheatgrass. Now, I had never done any of these before. The thought of needles being stuck into my body was a bit frightening; I could hardly stand to think about it. And royal jelly? Was I really prepared to ingest honeybee secretion? Plus, was pretty sure I was allergic to bees. And Fertility Yoga sounded so woo woo. At the time, I was such a rookie to all of these naturopathic treatments, I didn't know what to make of it all. But I was willing to try. I was willing to do anything.

The first thing I did was book myself an acupuncture appointment. Fertility acupuncture works like this: the acupuncturist places needles at certain trigger points in your body to help direct the flow of blood to the uterus when your egg is developing. This in turn is supposed to drive more oxygen to the egg, which encourages it to grow bigger and more viable. That reasoning made complete sense to me.

On the Friday of my appointment, I casually mentioned to Samir the many success stories I had read of women with low AMH getting pregnant with the help of acupuncture. He was skeptical.

"I don't know about acupuncture. Isn't that a bit extreme?" he asked, as if waiting to see my reaction.

I decided not to tell him where I was headed that day. I could sense he wasn't into the idea, and I didn't want to let any negativity distract or dissuade me from trying acupuncture for the first time.

The practice I had found specialized in fertility acupuncture, and their office was located on Michigan Avenue. When I walked in, not a soul was there. The waiting room was completely empty. Finally, a woman came out and told me to fill out a form. I filled it out quickly and then waited. And waited. And waited. *What is going on here?* I thought.

About half an hour later, the woman came back and ushered me into a back room with a massage table laid out. She told me to undress, lay down, and then cover myself with the sheets. I did as she said and waited. Maybe I should have told my husband—or someone—where I was going.

After what felt like an eternity, the woman finally came back and started pulling out needles. I told her it was my first time trying acupuncture.

"Will it hurt?" I asked, looking for reassurance.

"Don't worry," she said. That was her only response. I felt like a child whose fears were being glossed over by a dismissive adult.

She then proceeded to prick and prod me with pins. Each one felt like a sharp pinch, a sensation that was more shocking than painful. Once all of the needles were in place, she left me to lay there for a half hour.

When she returned, she pulled out all the needles and said, "That's it."

I got dressed and collected my things.

This first brush with acupuncture was nothing like what I thought it would be. I had expected compassion and understanding—

or at least a practitioner who would take the time to explain the unfamiliar procedure to me. When I walked out of that appointment, feeling cold and empty, it was as if I didn't know what had just happened to me.

They say that acupuncture helps to release and purge the toxins in your body. But the experience left me queasy and shaken. Could one session have released that many toxins from my body to such extreme effect?

As I checked out at the front desk, the acupuncturist recommended weekly appointments to me, and I politely responded that I would call in and schedule them. I never followed up. In reality, I couldn't bear the idea of going back to that sterile room.

Fertility acupuncture and I did not get off to a good start, to say the least. But that did not deter me from giving fertility yoga a try. I knew there had to be something out there in the world of holistic fertility treatments that I could connect with.

I went to my first yoga class at Pulling Down the Moon, a holistic health center in Chicago, on a Saturday morning in July. The studio was decorated with portraits of Hindu gods, the Sanskrit letter for Om, and figures of Ganeshji that were familiar to me from growing up in an Indian household.

I could sense the collective mood of love and acceptance in the room as I grabbed a yoga mat and found a spot between the other women in the class.

Once the studio had filled up, the yoga teacher greeted us: "Good morning, ladies! Welcome to the first session of fertility yoga. We're going to start today by going around the room, introducing ourselves, and sharing why we're here. I'll start. My name is Kelsey. I'm here today because I believe in taking a moment for self-reflection every day. I know how personal it is to share your stories with me and a room full of strangers, so we will start slow. At the beginning of each class, we will form a circle just like this, and you can share as little or as much as you like. This is a safe space to share any updates, stresses, milestones, feelings of grief or hurt, and setbacks."

One by one, each of the women in the class introduced themselves, shared why they were there, and said a little bit about where they were in their fertility journeys. Our class had gathered people from all walks of life who were struggling with everything from endometriosis, diminishing egg quality, reoccurring miscarriages, to getting pregnant as a member of the LGBTQ community or having no clear answer at all as to what was impacting their fertility. The circle finally snaked its way back to me and then it was my turn to share.

"Hi, my name is Julie. My husband and I have been trying to get pregnant for over a year. My doctor has me on a Clomid and IUI treatment plan right now. We just had our second procedure and it didn't work, so I thought if I tried something different, it might help. That's why I'm here."

For the first time during the lonely struggle of trying to get pregnant, I felt at home. I was now a part of a community that understood what I was going through and was enthusiastically there to support me.

We spent the rest of the class working through beginner yoga poses on our mats. Since this was actually the first time I had ever attended a yoga class, even common poses such as Downward-Facing Dog and Cat-Cow were new to me. I took pleasure in learning them. Our main objective was to increase blood flow to the uterus. We stretched and positioned our bodies to reiterate and emphasize this goal.

The lights in the room had been dimmed. With only the light from a small candle burning at the front, it felt as though it was a little past dusk, instead of Saturday morning. Throughout the one-hour session, we held moments of silence where Kelsey guided us to relax, breathe, and reflect on our intentions. Mantras played in the background—the musical hymns I grew up listening to because my dad is a Hindu priest—which made me feel so at home. Every second of that class, I envisioned a tiny baby growing in my uterus. Oh, how I wished that I could truly make it happen.

By the end of our first session, I felt refreshed and energized—like I had been transformed into a new person and anything was possible. I was super woman; I could already feel the shift in my body on both a cellular and spiritual level.

The girls I met in yoga class changed my life. For the next six weeks, yoga became my happy place and refuge. I could hardly wait for Saturday mornings—even though it meant waking up super early—because it was the one time each week when I could be myself and share my innermost thoughts and deepest fears. I depended on my yoga sisters to get me through all the doctor's appointments and disappointments.

We were a tribe. Even though we were all so different, we shared the same pain. We shared our stories openly and honestly. With no fear of judgement. No patronizing advice. No disapproving looks. No assumptions. Just acceptance and support. We cried for one another when a cycle failed and cheered when we heard success might be around the corner for one of us. And I am sure that we all prayed silently that each of us would find our peace one day.

Looking back, the hour I spent in fertility yoga each week was one of the most cherished times of my life. Pulling Down the Moon also offered fertility acupuncture, which helped me give the treatment a second chance. It turned out they had one of the best acupuncturists around.

Lexi had studied at Pacific College of Oriental Medicine in New York City and had interned for fertility expert Mike Berkley. Before we began our first session, Lexi took the time to introduce herself and her background and then proceeded to listen to the struggles I had encountered thus far in the journey to getting pregnant. She explained how fertility acupuncture helps women to achieve and maintain pregnancy by enhancing healthy blood flow to and from the uterus.

I felt myself exhale when she said that. I had read so many success stories of women becoming pregnant through fertility acupuncture, and I truly believed it could boost all of the other treatments I was already undertaking—which is why my negative experience with it the first time around had been so crushing.

Lexi left the room while I undressed, and as I lay on the table waiting for her to return and begin the session, I felt completely at peace and surrounded by the most soothing aura. Maybe it was the gentle light emanating from the candle in the corner of the room, or

Lexi's tranquil and comforting energy, or maybe it was because I already loved the yoga classes at Pulling Down the Moon so much. Either way, I felt at home.

When Lexi returned, she explained which trigger points she would focus on and place needles in, and then proceeded to play a lilting mantra on a nearby speaker. I closed my eyes as she continued, barely noticing the needles going in. I focused on my breathing and the music. As she finished, she whispered that she would leave me to relax and come back in thirty minutes. I felt such an inner calm that I barely noticed her leaving, and before I knew it, the session was over. I was hooked and saw Lexi regularly for the next fifteen weeks.

Lexi and I became friends. I was beyond thankful for her expertise and compassionate bedside manner. I felt myself getting stronger, physically and emotionally, in her care. I was proud of the fact that I hadn't let myself quit. Finally, my stubborn determination seemed to be paying dividends, affirming that I was on the right path.

A few weeks into yoga class and the acupuncture treatments, I came home and caught the reflection of myself in our condo window. I felt invigorated and could see the undeniable transformation in my body. I was glowing—and I had never felt healthier or more alive. I smiled back at my reflection because I knew something had shifted and the world looked a bit brighter.

The next Saturday at yoga we sat in our circle to share updates as usual. Helen, who was an HR professional with blonde hair and sparkling blue eyes, broke the news that she and her husband were relocating. Before we could congratulate her on the move or tell her how much we were going to miss her, she turned to me and said she had one more thing to share.

"Last night I had a dream, and you were in it, Julie," she said, smiling. "You were pregnant. I know it's going to happen. I can't wait for reality to catch up with my dreams!"

I was so shocked and honored by this unexpected prediction. It felt like all the worrying, late-night googling, and lifestyle adjustments were finally paying off. Things were beginning to fall into place. I believed soon my baby would be too. I never let that thought fail me.

6
WHEATGRASS & OTHER EXPERIMENTS

Buoyed by my newfound support group at yoga, I continued to experiment with the naturopathic fertility treatments that were talked about in the online forums I visited regularly.

To kick my caffeine addiction, I replaced coffee with smoothies. I bought myself a Magic Bullet blender, added fruit, water, and mixed it all up. Any time I caught myself craving a cup of coffee, I made myself a smoothie instead.

I also started taking shots of wheatgrass—one to two tablespoons a day in a glass of lukewarm water—because I had read that it has cleansing properties and helps lower high FSH or follicle stimulating hormone that helps women ovulate. Women have a set number of eggs, which means the quantity decreases over time and ages with their bodies. Fewer eggs and lower overall egg quality trigger a woman's body to try and restart the ovulation process by increasing levels of FSH, which counterintuitively makes it even more difficult to conceive. By consuming wheatgrass, I could help reverse the effects of high FSH, as well as remove some of the toxins stored in my cells and prepare the body for pregnancy.

The only catch? Wheatgrass is one of the nastiest things I've ever tasted. Imagine eating a fistful of freshly plucked grass, roots with clumps of dirt and all, and that's exactly how it tasted—like drinking mud. Most of the time I just chugged the wheatgrass-water concoction and hoped it went down before I could fully taste it.

Not everything I tried was as hard to swallow, though. Royal jelly, a substance secreted by honeybee workers and fed to larvae and queen bees, made me skeptical at first but it was easy enough to add into my diet. Thick and soft, it was like eating honey that had been rolled up in a ball. The recommended dosage is one to two teaspoons twice daily. Royal jelly is quite literally a natural super food as it fuels the queen bee and nourishes her so that she can lay more than 2,000 eggs per day.

One fertility website explained that, "Royal jelly is rich in amino acids (29 to be exact), 10-hydroxydecanoic acid (10-HDA), lipids, sugars, vitamins, and proteins. It contains vitamins A, B complex (including folic acid and inositol), C, D and E, and also has ample levels of iron and calcium, as well as other minerals. Because royal jelly contains a wide variety of nutrients that are essential to proper health and organ function, it is very easy to see how it can help assist fertility."[1] If this sticky, sweet substance could help queen bees lay thousands of eggs a day, I figured it could assist me in creating at least one healthy human egg.

I also started taking maca root capsules, an herb that grows at high elevations in the Andes region of central Peru. For centuries, Peruvian locals have used maca as a food source (it's similar to broccoli and cauliflower) and treatment to increase stamina and energy. Recent scientific studies have shown that maca root supports hormonal balance and reproductive health for both males and females. The key phrase I looked for in all of these natural remedies was "reproductive health."

In addition to regular prenatal vitamins, I added in supplements like CoQ10 and DHEA. Coenzyme Q10 is a nutrient present in almost all cells that our bodies naturally produce. In fact, it generates 95 percent of the energy that keep our bodies functioning at the cellular level. The highest concentrations of CoQ10 can be found

---

[1] Hethir Rodriguez, "Fertility Super Food – Royal Jelly," Natural Fertility Info, December 14, 2018, https://natural-fertility-info.com/royal-jelly.html.

in the heart, where it aids the cardiac function. It also acts as a powerful fat-soluble antioxidant that protects against free radicals that lead to cell damage.

What that means in plain English is that CoQ10 stimulates cell regeneration and promotes healthy, functioning cells. I ordered 750 mg capsules of CoQ10 from Fertilica along with 100 mg capsules of Ubiquinol, the purest form of CoQ10, so that I could boost my body's natural cell regeneration process and fortify my remaining eggs. I took one of each capsule with meals daily.

I was more hesitant to try dehydroepiandrosterone or DHEA because my Google research turned up contradictory opinions. Many women raved about DHEA online and said it worked wonders for them. Considering the desperate situation I was in, I could hardly say no to trying something that had proven to be incredibly effective for other women trying to get pregnant.

But DHEA is not an herb. It's a steroid hormone created by the body from cholesterol in the adrenal glands and its occurrence in our bodies naturally decreases over time, reaching its peak during our mid-twenties. Most doctors and fertility groups don't support the use of DHEA supplements because it's not natural to have such high levels of DHEA in our bodies when we're older and it can lead to hormonal imbalance over the long term.

In the end, because I knew so many people attested to DHEA's ability to promote egg health in women, I decided on a compromise. I would take less than the recommended dosage. Instead of two 25 mg pills a day, I took one.

I was determined to do whatever was within my power to increase the likelihood of me getting pregnant. This quest began to consume nearly all of my energy and brainpower. Keeping track of all the supplements and herbs and spoonfuls of royal jelly and making sure I made it to all of my weekly appointments and classes quickly turned into a full-time job. At my real job, I was preoccupied, daydreaming about what it would be like to finally be pregnant, and just getting by doing the bare minimum. My heart wasn't in the work anymore.

My sudden and intense desire at thirty-eight to become a mother was all-consuming. I had tunnel vision, which was simply my way of working towards a goal I had set my mind on; I became obsessed with it. While the supplements and new health regimen were physically and chemically altering my body, the emotional and psychological journey I had embarked on was also changing me, Julie, on the level of my soul.

No one can ever prepare you for what your body will go through in the aging process. We each experience it differently, and it may be gloomy to look at it this way, but everyone suffers from some existential crisis sooner or later. Life leaves very few of us unscathed, whether it's fertility problems, chronic depression, late-stage cancer, or losing a loved one without whom we can't imagine living.

Getting pregnant when the odds are stacked against you requires every ounce of faith you can muster. We were several months in at this point and had no idea whether there was ever going to be a happy ending in sight. Sometimes the uncertainty overwhelmed me and stopped me in my tracks. *What am I doing? Who am I?* All I could do was hope that everything was going to make sense in the end. That it was all leading somewhere.

The yoga community at Pulling Down the Moon was such a boon to me in this respect because all of us there were living daily with the same uncertainty. I leaned on them to get me through a lot of tough moments.

Samir and I hadn't told either of our parents yet about the steps we were taking to conceive, even though I knew they were eager for us to give them grandchildren. I wasn't ready for the pressure that letting them in on our plans would entail, and I also wasn't sure they would understand the process in the first place.

Instead, whenever I lost it, I turned to my sister, Jalpa, or my best friend Reshma. Both were my sounding boards when I needed a second opinion. One day I called my sister as I was walking home from work. We had just failed another IUI and I was feeling pretty low. I told Jalpa how all of my friends were getting pregnant. Of course, I was genuinely happy for them, but at the same time, I was plagued by the nagging question: Why couldn't I do the same?

As I was walking and talking to my sister, I felt the pressure and expectations building up inside me. I was exhausted from all the meds and treatments—and the frustration of realizing that none of it was seemingly working. I felt so overwhelmed in that moment that I started crying.

"Julie, it's okay . . . . Take a deep breath," Jalpa said, trying to calm me down. "What does Samir say about everything?"

Although Samir didn't always understand what I was going through, he supported me absolutely, without question. A couple weeks before he had mentioned the idea of me quitting my job and taking some time off. I had envisioned myself leaving work to raise our children anyway, and we had long ago agreed that it was important to both of us that once we had children, I would stay home to raise them at least until they were school bound. We believed in taking a hands-on parenting approach to our family, as that is how we were both raised, and I was happy to take on this role.

"He says I can't worry about this so much," I answered. "He says it's okay if we can't have children. He still says we can travel and see the world, that we will be just fine." As I repeated Samir's words to my sister, I wondered, *My God, has he given up on the idea of having children?* This thought hadn't crossed my mind before.

Just then, a loud honk pulled me out of the conversation. I jerked my head up and saw a speeding car brake hard to avoid hitting me. Breaking free from my tunnel vision, I now noticed slack-jawed pedestrians stopping to stare. The driver, who was visibly shaken up, looked straight at me through his windshield. They were all trying to make sense of what I had just done and check that I was okay.

I was in shock. Absorbed by the thoughts racing through my head, I had walked off the curb onto a busy street, neither looking to check traffic nor stopping to realize the "Don't Walk" sign was lit up. I had nearly killed myself and could have injured others.

On the phone, still gripped in my hand, I could hear my sister, alarmed, "Julie! Julie, hello! What happened? Hello!"

*   *   *

When I got home, I nearly collapsed onto our couch. How could I have been so reckless? So thoughtless? I had reached my breaking point. I was supposed to be bringing new life into the world, not putting myself in danger. I decided not to tell Samir because I didn't want to alarm him. But I thought more seriously about what he had said about quitting. Initially, I resisted the idea because I thought that I could do it all—juggle work and the fertility treatments. It had become patently clear that I was overwhelmed by everything that was happening in my life.

Maybe taking some time off was not such a bad idea. I weighed the pros and cons in my head. Without the added stress of performing at work, I would have more time to rest and get in the right mind space. The meds and supplements could only do so much on their own; I doubted whether I could get pregnant if I wasn't also psychologically healthy.

But what if I quit and never got pregnant? Then what? Would I be able to get my old job back? I reminded myself of all that I had accomplished in my sixteen-year career. My resume spoke for itself. I could find another job if I had to. And I was grateful that our finances were grounded enough.

I slept on the idea for a few more nights, and then one Friday towards the end of July, I decided it was the day. I was nervous to tell my manager, who had become a friend. But I knew it was now or never. She sat in the next cubicle over, so I walked over to the printer to pick up my resignation letter, folded it into an envelope, then walked back to our cubicle area and tapped her on the shoulder.

"Hey Casey, do you have a minute?" I handed her the envelope. She opened it and just stared at it for a few seconds.

"Are you serious?"

After the initial surprise wore off, we went over to an empty conference room where we could talk. I hadn't told anyone at work about the fertility treatments Samir and I were going through. Broaching such deeply personal issues like infertility or miscarriage at work still felt taboo. It just wasn't done, even though it was 2013, not 1965. So I kept my explanation upbeat and vague: I was at a point in my life where I was ready to explore "other things." I thanked her for the opportunity.

Although I knew I had left Casey flabbergasted, handing in my resignation was such a relief. An aura of peace and calm settled over me, and I knew I had made the right decision. At lunchtime, I called Samir, who didn't know I had planned to quit that day, to tell him the news.

"Good for you, honey. I'm so proud of you," he said in a softer tone than his usual voice. I realized I hadn't heard him this content in a long time. Maybe I imagined it, but I think he breathed a sigh of relief.

I felt the weight of all the responsibilities I had been carrying melt away. We would take a trip to Napa to get away from everything in Chicago, and once we returned, I would be able to focus full time on nurturing my body and mind for the baby we hoped would arrive.

7

SIGNS & MIRACLES

The events of the past few months seemed to shrivel up and evaporate the moment I stepped on the plane for our trip to California in September. By the time we touched down at San Jose airport, I was in full vacation mode and pumped for our first night in the Bay Area.

Manish, one of Samir's good friends from college, was waiting at the airport to whisk us away to dinner at a trendy tapas restaurant, where his girlfriend Jana and one of Manish's coworkers would meet us. After dinner, we would head over to the night's main event: a Depeche Mode concert at the Shoreline Amphitheater.

We were filled with excitement since we were going to see our all-time favorite band from high school. Samir had been tracking Depeche Mode's Delta Machine world tour and saw that they were playing in Northern California, which was the perfect excuse to finally visit Manish and Jana.

At Shoreline Amphitheater, which is a beautiful, outdoor concert venue in Mountain View, we found a central spot on the grass with a good view of the stage and laid out a blanket for us to sit on. As people kicked back beers, I breathed in the fresh mountain air. I watched the sky metamorphose into a bright orange streak with bursts of yellow and pink before finally melting into the blues and indigos of twilight. Chicago and what our lives had become there felt like a distant planet.

Once the stage lights dimmed, the crowd began to murmur with anticipation, until the cheers rose to full volume, with people whistling and hollering. Finally, the shadowy outlines of the band appeared on stage, their figures cutting through the clouds of smoke that had been pumped out for dramatic effect. We all burst into shrieks of elation, and before I knew it, Dave Gahan's familiar voice enveloped the amphitheater and we were on our feet dancing. Boy, did we dance. It reminded me of our first date at The Fray concert.

An hour and a half into the show, Depeche Mode started banging out their greatest hits and their performance wound its way towards its climax. The crowd was enthralled with nostalgia, us included, as we relived the moments that iconic songs like "Just Can't

Get Enough," "Personal Jesus," and "People Are People" conjured up from our collective pasts. I squeezed Samir's hand when I heard the first bars of "Somebody" and he pulled me into an embrace.

"I want somebody to share, share the rest of my life . . . Someone who'll stand by my side," Martin Gore sang. The words took me back—we had danced to the song for our first dance at our wedding —and it felt, for the moment, as though we had finally returned to the fun-loving duo we had always been. Samir and I needed this vacation more than we could have realized.

We slept in the next morning. The only thing that finally got us up was the smell of breakfast wafting from the kitchen, which became too tempting to ignore. As we walked upstairs from the bottom floor that Manish and Jana had generously let us take over, I couldn't get over how glorious the views were from each and every window in the house. We were surrounded by majestic, golden mountains.

After we finished eating breakfast, Jana offered to take us for a drive down the 17-mile coastline of Pebble Beach. The landscape was absolutely breathtaking. On one side of the car were the foothills peppered with tall, weather-worn cypress trees, and on the other side was the ocean as it crashed against stretches of beach and jagged, rocky cliffs. We stopped for several photo ops along the way.

Our vacation skated by in this breezy way, with every day spent in the replenishing presence of nature and sunshine and good company. It was fun getting to know Jana and see the loving relationship that had blossomed between her and Manish. Hanging out with them was so easy and laid back, it was like being with family. I could see how happy they were together, which seemed like the first step toward a glowing future.

On our last day of the trip, the four of us headed north to Napa Valley for a day of vineyard hopping. Since I had taken the month off from IUI treatments, wine was not off limits. Bring on the tastings!

Jana, ever our consummate host, acted as our tour guide for the day. We started at Domaine Carneros, a vineyard that has the aura of a French chateau with the extravagant architecture and manicured rose gardens to match. This particular winery is known for its sparkling wine and Pinot Noir, so we sampled a little of both. Before moving on with our day, I made a trip to the ladies' room and while I was in there, I noticed there was a bit of blood on my underwear. The spotting was a bit odd because it was too early for my period, but I didn't linger on it and rejoined everyone without a second thought. Then we were on to our next stop: Artesa, a vineyard established by Spain's oldest winemaking family. It had a more rustic feel to it that I appreciated in contrast to the pomp of Domaine. The best was still yet to come.

At Sterling Vineyards, which sits at the top of a hill, the only way to get there is via an aerial gondola. We lifted into the air and the rows of grape vines beneath us transformed into an abstract pattern of green, bushy lines as far as the eye could see. The rolling hills all around us were sun-kissed in the late afternoon light.

Once we had tasted our fill of fine wines, we ended the day with dinner at an Italian restaurant in town. With our tummies full and hearts happy, we thanked Manish and Jana for a wonderful vacation and told them they should come visit us in Chicago soon.

The next morning we flew back. Once we were settled at home, I threw myself into pulling together the finishing touches for the baby shower I was co-hosting for Shaila. Her sister had taken the lead in planning the party and her good friends, Jasmine, Anu, and I were helping out in whatever ways we could. We wanted the shower to reflect the personalities of Shaila and her husband Mischa, who made a pastime out of sampling food and wine together, so we booked Terzo Piano at the Art Institute of Chicago. The restaurant, which is housed in the modern wing of the museum, has clean lines and modern silhouettes with floor-to-ceiling windows and incredible views of the city.

On Saturday afternoon, the day of the shower, we were a lively group of ladies lunching and chatting in our own partitioned-off area of the restaurant. The theme was "Ready to Pop." Kind of cheeky for a baby shower, but we had a lot of fun with it. We had tiny bags of popcorn tied with bows, cake pops, frosted sugar cookies with the word "pop" iced on them, and plenty of champagne to top off the theme. Mischa and Shaila wanted to keep the party gender-neutral since they didn't know the sex of their baby. And because Mischa is Dutch and a huge soccer fan, we made sure to use lots of orange, which is the Dutch national team's jersey color. The tables were decorated with vases of orange flowers and we had a few orange balloons floating around. Everyone was dressed to the nines in flowery frocks and heels; the four of us who had helped organize the party opted to wear our most festive orange outfits.

That party was a blast. We nailed the theme, and everyone loved it. I was so happy for Shaila and grateful to be a part of the celebration —yet at the same time there was a feeling of wistful longing tugging at my heart. I couldn't help but wonder what it would be like to be pregnant myself, to have my sister and friends throw a baby shower for me one day.

Shaila was one of the first in my friend group to embark on this next stage of life: motherhood. She and I went way back. Though she was originally from Dubai, Shaila and I had met in Chicago after college when we were just single twenty-two-year-olds struggling to make our way in the world. We went out together, shopped together, gossiped about work and strategized career moves, supported each other through the travails of dating in the city, and cheered each other on when we finally found partners to share our lives with. We had grown up together through fifteen years of friendship. And now, Shaila was finally on her way to becoming a mother. I was so proud of her.

After we finished lunch, we gathered our chairs around Shaila's table and played several games. For one of the games, we had to guess how big Shaila's stomach was and whoever guessed closest to the actual measurement won a gift certificate to Pops for Champagne, a champagne bar in Chicago. Then we played a game of matching pictures of celebrity babies with their parents. Eventually Mischa arrived and we got down to opening presents and eating cake.

As guests started to leave, we gave each woman a gift bag and a bracelet. The bracelets were made of orange ribbons strung with silver beads that had inspirational words for new mothers imprinted on them, each one a different phrase. When it was my turn to leave, Shilpa, Shaila's sister, selected a bracelet at random and tied it around my wrist. I turned the bracelet around to read what it said and I nearly gasped when I saw the words. "Best Mom." My heart wanted to leap out of my chest. Instead, I composed myself and looked up at Shilpa and smiled.

On Monday, when the excitement from the trip and the shower had finally settled down, I thought back to our last day in California at the wineries and was reminded of the blood I'd discovered. I suddenly realized that I hadn't gotten my period yet. In fact, I was three days late . . .

The baby-making process and all the fertility treatments had been so far from my mind while we were gone. And then coming back to the flurry of tasks that had to get done for the baby shower, I'd completely forgotten where I was in my cycle and hadn't even thought about it. Now I realized my period was late. My periods were never late; they always ran like clockwork. Was it really possible? Could I be pregnant? But how?

The thought sent an electric jolt—excitement and fear—ricocheting through my body. The only thing to do was take a pregnancy test. I had stockpiled a bunch of cheapie home pregnancy tests early on, the kind you can order online for only a few cents each. I must have had a box of at least fifty tests that I had been using throughout the IUI process whenever I thought (or daydreamed) I might be pregnant.

I went to the bathroom, pulled one out from my stash in the cupboard, and proceeded to follow the instructions (which I had memorized by then). Then I sat and waited. The test stick was like a magic wand that had the power to decide my family's fate. Waiting for that second line to appear, the one that would confirm I was indeed carrying a baby inside me, felt like the longest wait of my life. And then when it actually did appear, I couldn't believe it. I had been so preoccupied with getting pregnant for the last eight months, I wondered if I had finally cracked. Maybe I was hallucinating. I needed someone else to verify that what I was seeing was objectively true.

I called Samir, but got his voicemail. I told him to call me back ASAP. I called my sister next and told her the news.

"Oh my god. Oh my god," she kept saying. "Are you sure?"

"I don't know, I think so. The test has two lines!" I nearly shouted.

"Oh my god. Okay, hold on a second. I have to find someplace quiet." She was at work at Marklund, a nonprofit where I had also previously worked. I knew and was friends with many of her coworkers; she didn't want them to overhear our conversation, so she went into one of the stalls in the women's restroom.

"Do you think it's possible that this is a mistake? A faulty test?" I asked.

"Send me a photo of it. I want to see," she said. I used my phone to take a photo of the two lines and sent it to her. Then I waited with bated breath.

"Oh my god," Jalpa said after several seconds of silence. She sat in the bathroom stall with tears streaming down her face. "Julie, you're pregnant!"

8
TWO HEARTS

By the time Samir called me back, I had already called Dr. Coffman's office and scheduled an hCG test for the next morning.

"We're pregnant!!!" I blurted out as soon as I answered the phone.

"What? Oh my god. Are you serious?" Samir said in short, clipped phrases as if he could barely get the words out.

"Yes, can you believe it?" I replied.

"No. Did you take a pregnancy test?"

"Yes! And it's positive," I said, as I texted over the photo of the test results.

"This is the best picture I have ever seen, J." I readily agreed—it was the best picture I had ever taken.

"Okay, now what? Did you call the doctor?" Samir asked.

"I called Dr. Coffman's office and made an appointment for tomorrow morning," I explained.

"Oh my god. I can't believe it," Samir said again. "Oh my god, J. I love you so much."

Later that evening Dr. Coffman called to congratulate us and then walked me through the next week of tests I'd need to undergo to validate the results I had received at home. The tests would also make sure the pregnancy was proceeding normally. There was no doubt in my mind, though, that I was carrying a new life inside me. I had jumped headlong onto the pregnancy train.

At home, Samir told me that he was so surprised and ecstatic at the good news, he could barely concentrate on anything else at work for the rest of the day. In the words of Jack from the movie *Titanic*, he felt like he was the king of the world. That night we slept soundly for the first time in a long time, as if we had both silently exhaled after months of holding our breath for good news. Breathing in fresh air never felt better.

I got up early the next morning and headed to my morning appointment. The nurse drew my blood and sent it to the lab to test for human chorionic gonadotropin (hCG) or what is sometimes called the pregnancy hormone.

When a woman becomes pregnant, meaning her egg has been fertilized and then implanted in the uterus, the placenta begins to form and secrete hCG, which in turn tells her body to continue producing progesterone. HCG levels must be higher than 25 IU/mL to signal pregnancy and are supposed to double every 48-72 hours in order for the pregnancy to be viable. The results of the blood test measured my hCG levels at 540.4 mIU/mL, a healthy amount above the minimum.

Two days later I was back in the doctor's office to draw another blood sample. My hCG levels had more than doubled to 1202.6 mIU/mL over the course of 48 hours just like they were supposed to.

After months of IUI regimens, none of which were successful, life had thrown us a curve ball; we had finally conceived on our own without the help of cutting-edge fertility treatments. Somehow, one of my eggs was left behind, Dr. Coffman explained, and my body didn't ovulate when it was supposed to. Instead, I must have ovulated four or five days behind schedule, which had coincided with the night that Samir and I made love. And voila, that's how the egg was fertilized.

After the second blood test validated my pregnancy, I had lunch with Jankhana, who has always been more like a sister. She was also one of the few people I confided in early about the IUI treatments Samir and I were going through. We chatted over veggie rolls at NIU Sushi lounge, updating each other on our personal lives and news about mutual friends. It was still early on in the pregnancy, and I had been advised not to tell friends and family yet. By the time the bill arrived, I could hardly keep the happy secret to myself anymore. I told her the news, and Jankhana instantly started crying. As a mother herself, she knew how much this meant to me, how it would completely change my world. All she could say was, "Oh my god, oh my god, oh my god! I'm so happy for you, JP." She promised she wouldn't breathe a word to anyone.

Once we knew my hCG levels were doubling as they should, Samir and I shared the news with both of our parents and immediate family, including Samir's sister's and brother's families. We were so excited and knew that they had been secretly waiting, praying, and hoping for us to get pregnant and start a family of our own. The voices on the other end of the phone were exactly what we needed to hear—full of pure joy and excitement, as well as a few stifled tears. I'm pretty sure that both of our moms ran to pray to God for his blessings as soon as we got off the phone. Nothing could have shattered our happiness in that moment.

Dr. Coffman wanted us to come in for our first ultrasound the next day. During the appointment, I sat on the examination bed and Samir sat next to me, holding my hand as the nurse technician operated the ultrasound machine. Dr. Coffman stood by and watched the monitor; he was checking to see whether the embryo had implanted in the lining of my uterus. In some cases, what they call an ectopic pregnancy, the egg doesn't make it to the uterus and gets stuck in the fallopian tubes where it can rupture—creating a dangerous situation for the mother and baby.

Our eyes were glued to the monitor as Dr. Coffman took over for the nurse and repositioned the ultrasound wand. Finally, he turned to us and then pointed at a small mass on the screen.

"There it is. The embryo is in the sac," he said matter-of-factly.

The egg had successfully implanted in my uterine lining, just like it was supposed to. Samir and I were over the moon with happiness. The pregnancy we had been trying so hard to bring about, which seemed like it might never happen, finally felt like a reality. We had to pinch ourselves. Dr. Coffman was cautiously optimistic and advised us to make our next appointment to check for the baby's heartbeat at six weeks.

Most women don't usually discover they're pregnant until five or six weeks in, but because of my punctual cycle, I had realized something was off only three days after my missed period. I was a little over four weeks pregnant when we began doing the blood tests, which meant I had to wait another week and half before I could come in for the next ultrasound.

I spent most of that week and half in a blissful state of shock. I continued with the healthy lifestyle changes I had incorporated over the past year—yoga, acupuncture, royal jelly, mindful meditation, CoQ10 supplements, and even those nasty wheatgrass shots. Given the unexpected miracle of this pregnancy, I had to believe that all of those practices had significantly boosted our chances.

Waiting for the next appointment was interminable only because I was so impatient to get to the next check-in milestone. To pass the time, Samir and I had nicknamed the baby "Peanut" because the embryo was a small, peanut-sized shape on the sonogram.

For the most part, I felt great. I was in good spirits and good health, and eager to begin this next chapter of life as a mother. I was so thankful, beyond thankful, for our little miracle.

The following Monday at six weeks, Samir and I shuttled back to Dr. Coffman's office. We joked and smiled at each other while we waited for the doctor in the patient room. I was sitting on the examination bed again and Samir was in the chair next to me. Dr. Coffman and the nurse technician came into the room and greeted us, then got right down to business.

"Now let's see if we can find the baby's heartbeat," he said as the nurse technician pulled the ultrasound machine out.

We watched in silence as the nurse adjusted and readjusted the positioning of the ultrasound image. Everyone's eyes were focused on the monitor. I picked out Peanut almost immediately; the embryo had grown noticeably since the last time we saw it. After a minute or two, the doctor broke his gaze with the image, took off his gloves, and turned to us.

"There's no heartbeat," he said gravely.

"No, I'm sure there's a heartbeat!" I responded instantly, as if it were a reflex. "Can't you take another look? Maybe you just missed it."

"I know this is difficult to hear," Dr. Coffman began.

"There's a heartbeat. I know it," I cut in.

"Why don't we do this," he offered, "Come back in a few days and we'll do another ultrasound on a different machine."

"Okay, thank you, Doctor," Samir said.

"Can you print copies of the sonogram for me to take home?" I asked.

"Yes, I'll have the nurse make them for you. Now go home and try to rest up. I'll see you in a few days."

We stopped at the nurse's station on our way out to pick up the sonograms. Samir had been mostly silent during the rest of the visit. I could tell that he was thinking about what the doctor had said, turning it over in his head, considering what it would mean for us. That he had any doubts about the baby hurt me. I was 100 percent certain the doctor was wrong. Peanut had a heartbeat. Dr. Coffman simply couldn't find it. It was just too early.

Outside the doctor's office, Samir and I said goodbye. He was heading back to work while I returned home on foot. As I walked the familiar route, I steeled myself for what I saw as the next battle in this pregnancy: carrying the baby to term. We had come so far. Surely this miraculous baby was not brought into existence for nothing. Everyone makes mistakes, even doctors. They had simply gotten it wrong this time.

I spent the rest of the day scouring internet forums and mommy blogs for any shred of hopeful advice I could find. There were many stories from women who'd had similar experiences—"When I went in for my second ultrasound, the doctor couldn't find the baby's heartbeat. My husband and I were devastated." I held onto the ones that fit my convictions. Some women had experienced faulty ultrasounds, which were overturned by later ultrasounds. Others said six weeks could be too early; not all babies develop at the same rate.

In our living room, I spread out all the sonograms onto the coffee table. I held each one of them up to the light and brought out a magnifying glass to get a closer look. When that didn't work, I started taking pictures of the sonograms with my phone and then used the touch screen to zoom in on the images. Then I cross-referenced what I saw on my sonograms with the sonograms that other women had shared online.

By late afternoon, I had spun myself into a ball of anxiety and exasperation trying to find incontrovertible proof that my baby had a heartbeat. I felt sick and went into the bedroom to lie down. The next few days were going to be torture.

*   *   *

At six weeks and three days, I went in to see the doctor for a second ultrasound. This time by myself. Samir couldn't take anymore time off of work and, on some level, he had already begun to accept the reality of what might be. Me on the other hand, I was stubbornly convinced I would see the heartbeat this time. I told him not to worry, I would record the whole thing.

We went through the familiar routine: I put on a patient gown and laid down on the bed; Dr. Coffman came in and a nurse technician began to conduct the vaginal ultrasound. She spent a few minutes repositioning it and shifting the image on the monitor. I held my breath when the doctor turned to tell me what he saw.

"I'm sorry, Mrs. Patel. There's no heartbeat."

I was in utter and total disbelief.

"That can't be," I said.

"In cases like this," Dr. Coffman said gently, "your body should naturally reject the pregnancy since it is no longer viable. So let's wait and see what happens over the next few days. But if it doesn't, we'll have to give you medicine to induce a miscarriage."

"I can't do that," I said, anguished at the thought. "I don't want to . . . hurt my baby."

"I know how difficult this must be, but you need to start thinking about the future. You have a healthy uterus—we know that much is true from the way the embryo successfully implanted—and we need to protect it if you want to get pregnant again. If your body doesn't reject the fetus naturally, you are opening yourself up to infection and other complications that will make it difficult for you to conceive again. You don't want to put yourself in danger, do you?"

"No," I finally conceded. I heard what he was saying, but it was as if I wasn't really there. My brain wasn't processing the meaning behind his words. *This is not happening. This is not real.* I kept repeating in my head.

I got dressed and gathered my things. I walked out of the doctor's office, but as soon as the door closed behind me, I was overcome with a feeling of panic. I had forgotten to get the sonograms of the baby.

I turned around immediately and made my way back through the waiting room in a daze. It was a busy morning and the place was packed with women, other hopeful mothers, waiting to be seen. I somehow propelled myself to the front.

"Excuse me, excuse me!" I had to wave to get the attention of the harried woman at the reception desk. "I didn't get a photo, the sonogram of my baby. Please, can I just go talk to the nurse?"

The receptionist nodded and waved me away. I walked back into the hallway connecting the patient rooms and offices, roaming around until I finally spotted my nurse.

"I didn't get copies of my sonogram. Can you print them for me?" The nurse hesitated before answering and looked at me as if checking to see if I was still all there. I'm sure she thought I was crazy, but thankfully she kindly obliged my request and soon returned with a sheaf of sonogram pictures. I went home and called Samir as soon as I stepped inside our condo. He picked up on the first ring. When I heard his voice, I had to choke back tears.

"They still can't find a heartbeat," I finally managed to say.

Samir was silent. I continued and told him how the appointment went, the steps we'd need to take.

"I told Dr. Coffman," I said through sobs, "I'm not going to take anything to induce a miscarriage. I mean, I just don't believe it. What if there's a heartbeat in a few days?"

"J, look maybe you are right," Samir offered. "But we also have to listen to the doctor. He agreed to give you a few days, so let's take that time. But we have to be strong and logical. We can't risk your health or our ability to try again, can we?"

All I could do was cry. Samir, even though he too was still processing the news, was sensitive to my emotional outpouring. He knew better than to keep pushing me on this point.

"Why don't you try to rest and we will talk more when I get home, okay?"

"Okay," I said.

I spent several hours analyzing the pictures of my baby, taking pictures of the pictures with my phone and zooming in, just as I had after the first ultrasound. Despite all the evidence to the contrary, I was convinced Dr. Coffman was mistaken. We had been through so many trials—IUI treatments, detailed health regimens, sleepless nights, tears, prayers, wishes—I had to believe it was all for something. That it had brought about this miraculous conception.

I proceeded to update the rest of our immediate family throughout the day since many of them had left messages for us and were anxiously awaiting any news. My sister was devastated when I called to tell her what happened at my doctor's appointment. She spoke to her husband, my brother-in-law, about it as soon as we got off the phone since he is also an OB-GYN. She spared me from describing the conversations they had.

The science behind the absence of a heartbeat in an embryo is pretty clear, and doctors see this every day. Emotions take a toll on one's heart and mind, blinding you from reality. That is what happened to me. I had no clear view of what was happening inside me, biologically and emotionally. I wanted this baby so bad, I didn't think anything could stop it from happening. I spoke to my mother later that evening.

"Your father and I are praying for you and the baby," she said, "You know, you should get a second opinion." I could tell that she herself couldn't believe such a thing as the baby not having have a heartbeat. "You could ask Dr. Shaw. Actually, I could ask them. Let me talk to them. I'm sure they could refer you to another doctor." The Shaws were good family friends who had known me since I was born. I knew them as my aunt and uncle, and both were successful OB-GYNs.

After Samir's parents heard the news, they had a similar reaction. They proceeded to reach out to their OB-GYN contacts, without being too explicit about what we were going through. No one wanted this joy to be taken away from our family. I mulled over the idea of seeking a second opinion and brought it up with Samir.

"Why don't we just see another doctor? I'm telling you, there's nothing wrong with the baby."

"Julie, we need to listen to Dr. Coffman and do what he thinks is best," he said, making his best effort to talk reason into me.

"We'll wait and see then," I relented.

The next few days passed at a snail's pace. I hadn't experienced any of the symptoms the doctor described that would signal the onset of a miscarriage, which made me feel vindicated. The baby was fine.

One night, as Samir and I lay in bed together before falling asleep, he put his hands on the barely noticeable baby bump my stomach had formed and whispered to it: "C'mon, Peanut, grow, grow. You can do it."

*   *   *

Dr. Coffman called a couple days later to check in. He was clearly concerned that nothing had changed and my body still hadn't rejected the fetus.

"Mrs. Patel, the longer we let this go on, the greater the risk you're putting yourself in," he said sternly. "I understand what a difficult decision this is, so I will give you three more days. If you don't miscarry naturally in that time, we will have no other choice but to bring you into the office and vacuum the fetus out."

Reality was starting to dawn on me. There was nothing I could do except continue in this futile waiting game. It was already mid-November, the week before Thanksgiving, so I kept my idle hands busy by setting up our Christmas tree. Sure, it was a month early, but it was all I could do to keep my mind off the inevitable.

My sister and mother, sensing that things were not getting better, came over to spend the day with me. With some prodding, they got me to get dressed and presentable enough to go outside and take a walk by the park. We went to a nearby Subway for lunch, and since they wanted me to stay out of the house for as long as possible, we sat down and ate there. They watched as I nibbled pathetically at a veggie sandwich. I know they tried their best to soothe me, but I just couldn't shake the dreadful feeling of waiting for something terrible to happen.

As soon as they left, I went into the bedroom and lay down. It was evening, and Samir was still at work. In the dark room, I took out my phone and went to the Things Remembered website. With a few clicks, I ordered a Christmas ornament: an angel engraved with the words "Peanut Patel forever in our hearts" with the date "November 2013" on the back.

It felt so cold and dark in the apartment by myself. *This is what hopelessness feels like,* I told myself. I began sobbing into the pillows uncontrollably. How was it possible that all these months of struggling to get pregnant could end like this? It felt so unbearably unfair.

Then I stopped. In the midst of my wailing, something had started to happen. There was a familiar sensation in my abdomen. I was cramping and soon it grew into the worst pain I'd ever experienced. I knew exactly what it meant—I was having a miscarriage.

I immediately went into the bathroom and sat down on the floor. In a matter of minutes, there was blood and embryo and tissue everywhere. Traumatic as it was, I somehow had the wherewithal to heed the instructions Dr. Coffman had given me if I were to have a miscarriage. He said that if I was able to, I should collect as much of the embryo tissue as possible in a container and refrigerate it until I could bring it in to the office the next day. He wanted to test the tissue to see if there was anything we could learn from it or prevent for the next time.

I cleaned myself up and found a plastic bag and an old Tupperware container. With an air of solemnity, I scooped up the embryo that my body had expelled into the bag and then placed it gently into the container. It looked so unceremonious yet strange in the

Tupperware that I felt compelled to find some way to make it feel distinct, loved.

I remembered that during any puja or religious prayer, my father, who is a Hindu priest, always wore a red shawl. I thought by wrapping my baby in something red I could not only honor his life, but also help send his soul to eternal peace, wherever that may be. Suddenly, I had a frantic need for a red shawl. Of course, we didn't have any red pieces of cloth in our apartment. The best I could do was a Santa hat.

It was soft and velvety, and perfect, actually. I cut off the white pom-pom and slit the fabric in half until I had made a square piece out of it. I then layered the red fabric at the bottom of the Tupperware container and nestled the plastic bag with my baby inside of it. I don't think I will ever look at a Santa's hat the same way again. However, the gesture gave me solace. I remember thinking, through all that pain, that the soft fabric would keep my baby warm in the fridge.

To complete this informal ceremony of sorts, I decided to say the Gayatri Mantra, a prayer in Sanskrit that my mom taught me to recite before bed as a little girl. Gayatri is the mother of all scriptures. She is in every breath and all of our senses, and she protects and nourishes humanity. I said the Gayatri Mantra for our little Peanut whom we never got to meet. It was the only way I knew how to find solace; I did what I needed to do to move on.

Exhausted and emotionally drained, I went back into the bedroom to lie down. I felt different. Maybe I was in shock, but there were no more tears. In their place was an eerie sense of strength. Maybe I was happy my body did what it was supposed to; maybe I was happy I didn't have to induce a miscarriage; maybe I was just happy I was able to say a prayer and send my baby off peacefully in the privacy of my home. While I didn't know where the sudden sense of calm had come from, I knew one thing for sure. I was going to the doctor's office the next day and wait on any results for moving forward. I was clear on that.

A few more minutes passed in this swirl of thoughts. Then the condo door opened, and I heard Samir's familiar footsteps walk through the dark. He took off his shoes. I could sense him standing in the doorway to the bedroom, so I looked up from the sheets.

"It's done," I said.

Without saying a word, he lay down next to me and held me in a tight embrace I wished would never end.

9

LEARNING HOW TO LET GO

Waking up to reality the next morning was not easy. But I knew what I had to do. I took Peanut in the Tupperware wrapped in the red Santa hat to the doctor's office. When Dr. Coffman and the nurse finally came into the patient room to see me, they spoke to me gently and with compassion in their eyes. I could see how badly they felt. In their own way, they were hurting for me.

"Wow, this is so nice—the way you wrapped it up," the nurse said as I handed the container over to her. She may have experienced something similar with other patients, or she may not have. Either way, she was kind and gentle. The glint in her eye made me feel as if she somehow did understand my pain.

"We'll take it to the lab to be tested and send you the results," Dr. Coffman explained. "If there is anything to be learned from the miscarriage, we will incorporate that information next time. Until then, your body needs to heal. It's best if you take this time to rest and recover, and then you can come see us next month."

I was so exhausted that I couldn't muster the energy to speak. I simply nodded in response and then gathered my things to head home.

Samir and I cancelled all our plans that weekend. His uncle was hosting a family get-together, so we called to say we couldn't make it. We decided to skip out on a 40th birthday celebration for Surabhi, a mutual friend. Our absence was out of character—we always showed up to social functions and loved unwinding with our friends. People began to wonder whether something was wrong.

We each coped with the loss of Peanut in different ways. Samir went back to work on Monday morning and I stayed home. Thinking of it now, being home alone with nothing to do after such a traumatic event sounds quite depressing—and I was deeply depressed about the miscarriage—but I wanted to be alone. I needed that time and space to process everything that had happened.

I called a few close friends over the next couple of days to tell them the bad news and get it over with. It's a painful and uncomfortable conversation; no one really knows what to say when you tell them you've had a miscarriage. Besides those limited and controlled contacts, I avoided people for the most part. I was still overcome with emotions: sadness, anger, frustration, desperation. I didn't want to be seen crying out in public.

Secretly, I envied Samir's ability to throw himself into work. At least he could keep busy and his mind off what had happened. What I didn't realize at the time was that it wasn't really easy for him either. Although he showed up to work every day, he was a shadow of himself. He roamed the halls of his office aimlessly, thinking about little Peanut, still not wanting to believe it was true. He felt more alone at work where his co-workers were oblivious to what was going on in his personal life. Back then (and even today in many cases) miscarriage was a stigmatized topic too sensitive to bring up at work, so he kept up the facade of professionalism and a stiff upper lip.

On Monday afternoon, Dr. Coffman's office called to tell me the results of the tests on the embryo tissue. The baby was a boy. Peanut was our precious baby boy. The tests determined that he had an extra X chromosome—a chromosomal defect that meant he never would have survived. I learned that it's actually one of the most common chromosomal disorders and was not something we could have prevented. Peanut's destiny was determined as soon as sperm met egg. There was nothing we could have done to save the pregnancy. It was

God's will. Knowing that didn't take away the pain of losing Peanut, but it allowed me to accept the fact that I had done everything I could to give this pregnancy a fighting chance. And that gave me some sense of closure.

The test results also made it clear that the miscarriage had not been caused by improper blood flow, inadequate uterine lining, or endometriosis—conditions that make it difficult for many women to carry a pregnancy to term. From the doctor's perspective, this was reason to be optimistic about the future. He reiterated his earlier instructions and said I should focus on recovering for at least a month. We still had time to try again.

I found comfort and support, as I had so many times before, in the online mommy and pregnancy forums that had become a fixture of my life over the past year. I read through dozens of stories from other women about their miscarriages, which helped me feel less alone. Many of the women focused on the silver lining that despite having miscarried, they were able to carry later pregnancies to term on the second, third, or even seventh try. I grasped onto that sliver of hope so tightly. I think, in the end, that's what brought me back to myself. As much as the loss of Peanut pained me, I knew I had to focus on getting better, on healing my body and mind so that we could try again.

*   *   *

Thanksgiving Day was exactly one week after the miscarriage. I woke up that morning and almost couldn't get out of bed. It was as if the weight of my depression had literally pinned me down to the mattress. The trauma and heartbreak were still fresh. Ready or not, Samir and I knew we couldn't spend the whole day hiding out from our friends and family.

Every year it's tradition for Samir's close-knit group of friends from college to get together for Friendsgiving, an annual event that people take turns hosting and something that we usually look forward to. Normally, I'm the person who finds any excuse to celebrate and throw a party. Not this year. The thought of facing so many friends and having to put a smile on my face, while inside I was still coping with this devastating loss, made me nauseous.

That morning, I put my phone on silent and didn't pick up or respond to any of the calls and messages from people who knew about the miscarriage—not even our parents, siblings, or close girlfriends. I knew any familiar voice would set off a chain reaction of emotions. The well-intentioned check-ins and questions of "Are you okay?" would have cracked me open like a broken fire hydrant and unleashed a never-ending stream of tears. I just couldn't go there. Even a simple "Happy Thanksgiving" would have set me off, and I still had the rest of the day to get through.

By sheer force of will, Samir and I filed ourselves into the car and drove away from the city and into the Chicago suburbs. We sat in silence for the entire 35-minute car ride. I fought tears back the whole way there.

As we parked outside Sudhir and Sonia's house, the friends that were hosting this year, I pulled down the sun visor on the passenger side and opened the mirror on it so that I could quickly touch-up my watery eyes. I took a deep breath and hoped that no one would notice.

Sonia opened the door with an enthusiastic, "Happy Friendsgiving, guys! Come on in," followed by a big hug. It took everything in me not to break down right there and then. Greetings from the rest of the gang soon rang out. Manish and Jana had flown in from San Jose for the holiday, and Tina and Kaushal, who also lived in the city, were there, as well as many other friends. None of them knew about the miscarriage, so the day would be strictly social—neither Samir nor I planned on bringing it up.

I tried my best to keep an upbeat attitude throughout the rest of the day and enjoy being among friends again, chit-chatting about frivolous things. Someone handed me a wine glass, and I didn't refuse since I knew it would be a while before we could start actively trying again. We snacked on appetizers—stuffed mushrooms, pasta salad, and

Indian curry—while the Turkey Day bowl games played in the TV room downstairs, where the guys had gathered almost immediately.

When dinnertime rolled around, we sat down to a catered feast with all the classic Thanksgiving Day dishes: stuffing, sweet potato gratin, green bean casserole, macaroni and cheese, mashed potatoes and gravy, and of course, a giant turkey. The spread was more than enough for the twenty or so guests. Dessert followed with several kinds of pies and ice cream on the side.

Even though I had dreaded it, once I was there, surrounded by friends telling stories and laughing about the good ol' days, I began to feel like myself again. I had finally regained my appetite, and boy, did I enjoy myself. At the end of the night when Samir and I got in the car and drove back to the city, our stomachs were heavy with food and our hearts a tiny bit lighter.

A few days later we met up with Manish, Jana, Tina, and Kaushal, this time at a sports bar downtown, so that we could all hang out with Manish and Jana one more time before they flew back to California. While the guys were glued to the television sets behind the bar and watching one of the weekend's big football games, us ladies settled into a seating area on the other side of the room where things were less rowdy.

Having been through the ordeal of Thanksgiving Day, I was feeling a lot stronger. I was ready to talk about the miscarriage, so I decided to break the news to Jana and Tina.

"So . . . ," I began while shooting them a tentative glance, "Samir and I got pregnant, but we had a miscarriage."

"Oh, Julie," Tina said with sympathy in her eyes, "I'm so sorry." Tina and Jana both hugged me and a few tears escaped from my eyes. I told them everything—how hard we had been trying to get pregnant, how excited we were when we found out we had done it naturally, and then the agony of waiting to see whether I would miscarry when we discovered there was no heartbeat. It felt good to finally talk about it, to have it out in the open and not have to pretend that everything was fine. Tina and Jana were so supportive. Jana told me not to lose hope, that there was no way the Julie she knew was not going to become a mom someday. While I knew things were more complicated than that, her words were encouraging and made me feel hopeful.

We got so involved in the conversation among the three of us, that I hadn't noticed how much time had passed. At some point, I finally looked up and saw that the bar had mostly emptied out. That's when I noticed Samir from across the room. He was slumped over with his head resting on Manish's shoulder and shaking so vigorously that at first I thought he might be laughing, as if the guys had cracked some hilarious joke. But it wasn't that at all. Samir was crying. Not just crying, but sobbing—like a little boy—and I could hear his wails clearly now. I felt my heart spasm.

The guys, just like the ladies had done for me, were there supporting Samir, doing what friends do. They were listening to Samir's pain, giving him a chance to let it all out, and at the same time, trying to soothe his worst fears and give him something to hope for. Kaushal rubbed Samir's back and gave him a hug.

The ladies and I watched for a minute or two to let the guys have this moment together before crossing over to the bar. I put my arm around Samir and we embraced. Our closest friends now understood the depths of what we had suffered in silence and it was a huge relief. Samir and I had tried so hard to keep up a brave face in public, it almost did us in.

But now that the unspeakable had been spoken, our friends rallied around us. Everyone began sharing stories of friends and acquaintances they knew who had gone through miscarriages or struggled, sometimes years, to get pregnant. It turned out we were not alone at all. There were people within our own close-knit friend circle who had experienced similar challenges. Social norms had kept us from opening up to each other and sharing these stories publicly, but with this new perspective, Samir and I were able to realize that these things happen to everyone.

We had pillars of strength that were ready to hold us up, and a tribe of people around us who had experienced similar heartache and loss. Why wasn't anyone talking about their experiences? Samir and I felt so much lighter after opening up, sharing our grief, and realizing we were not alone. Everyone should have a platform where they can open up like that. Miscarriage is not something to be ashamed of. It is a loss of a baby, and it should be openly grieved and talked about as such. It turned out that Thanksgiving was the catalyst we needed to kickstart the healing process.

*   *   *

November quickly turned into December. I received an invitation from Surabhi who was continuing her 40th birthday celebrations with an all-girls trip to Cancun. I told Samir I wasn't going, that the timing was just too soon. To my surprise, he urged me to reconsider.

"J, I think you should go," he said gently. "You know, it could be really good for you to get away for a few days. Clear your head and relax."

Nothing was going to happen in December anyway, I realized, since the doctor had given me strict orders to rest and recover. He wasn't even going to entertain the conversation of starting IUI treatments again until the new year.

"You're right. What the hell, I'll go to Cancun and get a tan!"

A day later, I had booked my flight and splurged on a single room at the resort that we'd all be staying at. The other ladies would be bunking up and sharing rooms, but I figured I could use the space and solitude to decompress in between birthday activities.

The resort in Cancun was a sight to see when we arrived there after more than four hours of travel. The entrance was all decked out for Christmas with beautiful glass ornaments and lush, tropical garlands to reflect the local flora and fauna. We were greeted by staff in the lobby with trays of cocktails that looked like mini sunsets captured in a glass. My room had an incredible view of the ocean below. I opened up the windows immediately to let in the fresh salt spray.

The next few days were filled with massages and margaritas, sunbathing and gabbing with the girls as we took dips in the pool. Every night, we got dressed up in our colorful, vacation-ready outfits and sat down to sumptuous dinners with ocean views. The trip was a blast. Being able to retire to my own bed every night after such fun outings with the girls and luxuriate in the queen bed I had all to myself with 700-thread-count sheets was a dream—just what the doctor ordered.

Samir had been so right. I arrived back in Chicago in time for Christmas, feeling refreshed and renewed. This time when I looked at the special ornament we had made for Peanut, any sadness I felt was eclipsed by the overwhelming and immense feeling of love and gratitude that now flowed through me. I knew that Samir and I still had so much love to give and that we would have another chance to try again, hopefully soon.

10
SECOND CHANCES

Samir and I had made a conscious effort during the December holidays to slow down and appreciate the simple pleasures in life —whether it was enjoying a glass of wine with friends, gathering for Christmas meals and gift exchanges with our families, or just snuggling into the couch together to watch movies on Netflix. We gave ourselves the space to reflect on the trauma we'd been through. The realization that we weren't alone in the struggle to get pregnant—that many of our friends, in fact, had faced similar challenges—grounded us, gave us the ability to call upon a strength we didn't know we had.

When the new year rolled around, I was ready to jump back into the game and start fertility treatments again. I went back in to see Dr. Coffman the first date he was available in January. He seemed happy to see that I was in a much better state of mind since the last time we spoke. A doctor-in-training was shadowing him that day, so the three of us headed into a conference room and sat down.

For the benefit of his trainee, we went over the entire history of my treatment: the principle problem I faced was low AMH and decreased egg viability; I had gone through several rounds of treatment with Clomid and IUIs, all of which had been unsuccessful; I had completely overhauled my health regime with supplements, yoga, wheatgrass, and acupuncture; and what happened when we got pregnant naturally and didn't find a heartbeat. The miscarriage had been painful but necessary given the X chromosome defect. At the very least, it confirmed that I had a healthy uterus lining, which suggested we could be successful with a future pregnancy if we kept trying.

I had to stop myself from tapping my fingers on the table as the doctor walked through my fertility history. I squirmed in my chair, crossing and recrossing my legs. I knew it all too well and was impatient to get up to the present so that we could talk about next steps.

"Julie," Dr. Coffman finally turned to me, "Now that you've had a month or so to rest, how are you feeling?"

"I feel great!" I said, almost too enthusiastically. I figured I stood a better chance of getting the doctor to agree to begin treatments again if he saw that I was in good spirits. "The miscarriage was difficult to recover from, emotionally, but we had a lot of love and support from family and friends. Samir and I are ready to try again."

"That's wonderful. It sounds as though you are exactly where you need to be. Why don't you make an appointment to come back and see me in one month."

What? I had to wait another month before we could get started again? No, that was not what I wanted to hear.

"But . . . uh, Dr. Coffman, isn't there something we can do now?" I interjected. "I want to get pregnant again and I feel that time is of the essence. Maybe we can try IVF?"

"Whoa, whoa. Slow down," the doctor said with an unhurried calm that counteracted my frantic energy. "You've been through a major event—a miscarriage—and your body, as well as your heart and mind, is still recovering. We need to see what your body is doing before we start giving you more drugs or doing new procedures." He paused and put his hand on my shoulder, as if to transfer some of his own tranquil vibes over to me and soothe my nerves. "I know it feels like time is running out, but trust me. These things happen in mysterious ways and sometimes doing nothing for a period of time is the best medicine."

I looked at him doubtfully and sighed. I knew this wasn't a battle I could win with Dr. Coffman. Besides, he was probably right.

"Okay," I relented. "I trust your judgment."

"Come in on day three of your next cycle and we'll take a look, hopefully get you started on Clomid again, and give the IUI another try. In the meantime, you and Samir can certainly try on your own. How are you feeling right now? Let's see where you are in your cycle. You actually might be mid-cycle," he continued, as he looked through his charts and calendar. "Do you feel like you're ovulating?"

I had become so accustomed to listening to the rhythm of my body that I felt totally in tune with my cycle.

"Yes, actually I do feel like I'm ovulating."

"Okay," he nodded, "Why don't we go have a look on the ultrasound?"

I brightened up immediately at these words. Although Dr. Coffman had been firm about not beginning fertility treatments right away, he was always sympathetic to his patients' wants and needs. This was his low-key way of humoring me and giving me something positive to focus on.

The three of us moved into another room and the trainee set up the ultrasound machine. It didn't take long to see that there was indeed a follicle with a developing egg inside, about 14 mm. An egg should grow about 2 mm every other day and is considered healthy and viable once it reaches 16 mm.

"You will probably complete ovulation this weekend," Dr. Coffman advised, "So that would be a good time if you want to try naturally. Alright?"

"Thank you so much, doctor. We'll give it a shot." Despite having huffed and puffed about not being able to get back on a treatment train that day, I left the doctor's office feeling optimistic.

That evening when Samir came home, we ate dinner together. I told him about my trip to the doctor that morning.

"He doesn't want us to start fertility treatments until next month," I explained, "but we checked, and I'm ovulating. So we can try to get pregnant naturally. What do you think? I mean, we might as well give it a shot."

"Sure, let's see what happens," Samir said. Over the last year we had learned that starting a family would not be the sprint to pregnancy that we thought it was. This was a marathon, which meant we had to try every chance we got when the odds would be in our favor. Our eyes were locked on the prize.

We spent all day Sunday enjoying each other's company, beginning with a leisurely brunch and a stroll through downtown Chicago. *The Wolf of Wall Street* had recently come out, so in the afternoon, we went to see it in theaters. The film was intense. Watching Leonardo DiCaprio, one of my favorite actors, play Jordan Belfort, a brilliant but crooked, egotistical banker, was such a thrill ride. It really got my adrenaline pumping. Samir and I both loved it.

After the movie, we curled up at home, fully relaxed and rested. We were both focused on Sunday night thoughts—Samir was prepping for work the next day, and I was going over my plans for the week ahead. The thrill and rush from *The Wolf of Wall Street* was still fresh in our minds. We snuggled in bed and made love that night. For the first time in a long time, it felt completely natural and unplanned.

*   *   *

On Monday, we went back to our normal routine. I was back at yoga and taking all of my supplements every day. Samir was busy at work with a new project. After about two weeks, the day I was supposed to start my period rolled around. I was eagerly counting down the days so that I could make my next appointment with Dr. Coffman on Day 3. But the day came and went. No blood, no cramps, no period symptoms at all.

I was cautious not to read too much into this, even though I knew how consistent my cycle usually was. The last thing we needed was another false alarm to raise our hopes and then dash them. In the past, I would have been taking at-home pregnancy tests days before my period was supposed to start. This time I had the restraint not to test at all. I didn't even mention it to Samir. I was so nervous and scared about the possibility of being pregnant again that I didn't want to broach the subject, not with a ten-foot pole.

So I waited. A day or two into my missed period, Samir and I decided to unwind one night by taking a dip in our condo's pool. As we were walking out of our apartment, Samir grabbed a bottle of wine and started to reach for glasses in the cupboard.

"Do you want some wine when we get up there?" he asked.

I hesitated for a moment.

"Nah . . . none for me tonight," I said, trying to be nonchalant about it.

Samir shrugged. I could tell he thought my refusal was a bit odd, but he didn't push me on it, and we went on our way up to the pool.

I waited about a week before I mentioned anything to Samir. By this time, more than seven days had passed since I was due to start my period.

"I didn't want to tell you this until I was sure," I said to Samir at dinner that night. "But it's been a week since I was supposed to get my period. And I haven't had any symptoms either."

"Hmmm. So that's why you didn't want to drink wine the other day!" he said with a smile. "What should we do? Have you taken a pregnancy test yet?"

"I don't want a repeat of last time. That's why I waited to tell you."

"I understand, J. This has been rough on both of us. But we need to know the results, whatever they may be. Do you want to take a test now?"

I got out my stash of pregnancy tests and took one of them into the bathroom with me. When I finished, I left it on the bathroom counter and set an alarm for ten minutes before sitting down with Samir in the living room. Ten minutes was much longer than the recommended wait time, but I didn't want to take any chances. We waited anxiously for the time to pass. I felt as though I could hear the clock on the wall tick-tocking every single second in slow motion.

I actually had felt a change in my body. I felt pregnant and I knew it. But I wouldn't let myself entertain that thought too seriously, much less utter it aloud to Samir. I didn't want to do anything that could jinx a possible pregnancy.

When the buzzard finally rang, I was too scared to go back into the bathroom and check for myself, so I sent Samir instead. I clasped my hands together and closed my eyes as I listened to the sound of his footsteps lightly pad down the hallway to the bathroom. Then silence for several seconds.

"Well?" I yelled down the hallway anxiously. I opened my eyes and saw Samir running towards me out of the bathroom.

"There are two lines! We're pregnant!" he shouted, overjoyed. "You're pregnant!"

*   *   *

Samir and I celebrated the test results with hugs and kisses and tears. He was elated and I was relieved that my gut feelings had been validated. Since we were now five weeks into the pregnancy, one week further into the pregnancy than the last time when we had tested too soon, I was hopeful the blood tests and scans at the doctor's office wouldn't be as heartbreaking.

I called the office the next day and could barely get my words out as I gave the secretary my name and information. I explained that I had taken a pregnancy test the previous night. "There were two lines, so it looks like I might be pregnant. What do I do next?" I said this as if I had never been through the process before, even though in actuality I knew every step, inside and out. I probably could have explained it to her.

The secretary told me to hold on, she wanted to see if the doctor was available to get on the phone. I was sure she knew exactly who I was by that point—she and the other nurses had answered my calls enough times and complied with my requests for copies of ultrasound results. My emotions were high. I was nervous, excited, and scared all at the same time.

When Dr. Coffman got on the phone, he said congratulations. But I could tell he was cautiously optimistic. That was his usual response, supportive but realistic, which I had always appreciated. He scheduled the required blood tests, and I went in twice that week, 48 hours apart, to draw blood. The results came back positive; my hCG levels were doubling the way they were supposed to. Excitement was building up inside us again with each test result that confirmed the pregnancy.

The next test—and the point where everything went wrong for us last time—would be the ultrasound to confirm the baby's heartbeat. It was scheduled in one week, when I would be six weeks along. Every day I prayed like I had never prayed before. I was practically begging. "Please, God, give us this baby. We will love and cherish him or her for the rest of our lives."

The following weekend we had plans to celebrate a friend's 40th birthday up at Lake Geneva with our usual crew of friends. Based on past experiences, we had learned not to put our lives on hold. I needed to keep in touch with reality this time as best I could. Although a bit of a dicey move, we scheduled the ultrasound for Friday morning right before we planned to leave. If the news was bad, we would cancel and stay back in Chicago. That was the worse case scenario.

We packed for Lake Geneva Thursday night and the next morning, Samir and I went together to the doctor's office. Everything felt routine and familiar since we had done this before. I got undressed, put on the patient gown, and laid down on the examining bed. The nurse technician got the ultrasound machine ready. Samir sat next to me, holding my hand. I felt prepared for whatever results we might get, but as soon as Dr. Coffman walked into the room, a wave of nervous energy washed over me. This was it.

"How are you feeling?" Dr. Coffman asked after he sat down.

"Ready!" I said, and we all chuckled a bit, cutting the tension in the room.

"Good. Let's see what we have here."

Since I was at six weeks, Dr. Coffman conducted a vaginal ultrasound—they are the most accurate this early on. All eyes were on that grainy, blue and black screen as he began positioning the ultrasound wand. He readjusted it and then paused for a moment as he studied the image in front of us. He pushed a button on the machine and we heard a loud thump-thump-thump fill the room. I've never heard anything more beautiful.

I felt Samir grab my shoulder as my eyes filled with tears. I looked at the doctor and he said, "Yes, yes! That's it." His excitement followed on the heels of ours and his joy was undeniable. I looked at Samir and all he could say was, "Oh my god, oh my god! Yes."

"Do you see this flicker?" Dr. Coffman asked, helping to deconstruct the image on the screen. "That's the heartbeat. It is strong and healthy coming in at 108 beats per minute, which is a completely normal rate."

I couldn't believe what I was hearing or seeing. My heart stopped for a second as I watched my little baby's heart beat away.

I called my sister right after the appointment to tell her what we had witnessed; her words were practically inaudible as she tried to congratulate us. She was beyond overjoyed. We left the doctor's office elated, with the wind at our backs, as we hurried home. Tina and Kaushal would be picking us up soon for the hour-and-a-half drive to Lake Geneva. Samir and I agreed not to say a word to our friends. The happy news was just for us for now. If anyone asked why I wasn't drinking, I'd simply say I was on antibiotics.

Tina and Kaushal were their usual cheerful selves when they pulled up to our apartment building. Samir and I jumped in the back seat of their car and away we went for a weekend at the lake. The next few days would be filled with birthday activities: a spa day for the ladies, a private chef's dinner, and letting loose with a group of close-knit friends.

Samir reached over and squeezed my hand. Without saying a word, we looked at each other and smiled.

*   *   *

At the beginning of March, several friends asked how I wanted to celebrate my birthday since it was coming up on the 13th. We settled on the idea of doing afternoon tea at The Lobby inside the Peninsula Hotel.

Outside of immediate family, Samir and I had kept the secret growing inside my belly to ourselves. When we passed the 10-week mark, I went in to Dr. Coffman's office to do a MaterniT 21 PLUS test to screen for any chromosomal defects and determine the sex of the baby. We didn't want any surprises. Thankfully, the results did not turn up any abnormalities and we also found out we were having a baby girl! We were beyond elated and counted our blessings over and over.

It was getting harder to keep quiet about the pregnancy, not to mention my protruding tummy, so I hatched a plan.

On the day of my birthday tea, I arrived at the Peninsula with a stack of sealed cards gingerly packed into my handbag. I threaded my way through the elegant tearoom to a quiet corner in the back where

Tina, Shaila, Jankhana, Jasmine, and all the girls were seated. They had decorated the table specially for the occasion.

Three-tier serving trays filled to the brim with tea sandwiches—various combinations of cucumber, cream cheese, ham, salmon—were brought to the table. We each got to pick our own tea, which was then served in individual tea pots. The smell of fresh scones was almost irresistible; we wasted no time slathering them with jam and clotted cream.

We were all having such a lovely time, it finally felt like the right moment to share the joy that had filled up my life over the last several weeks. I dug into my purse to pull out the envelopes and began passing them out by name.

"What's this?" Shaila asked with sudden curiosity.

"Just a little something to thank you all for putting together this tea and being such good friends," I explained, a hint of mischief in my eyes. The table went quiet as everyone tore open their envelopes and read the cards silently. Inside each card I had written the same message:

Dear Masi,
    Thanks for taking my mom out for her birthday.
I'll see you all in October.
Love,
    Baby Patel

Masi means "aunt" in my native language, Gujarati. Each card was a message of gratitude from my future baby girl to her loving aunties.

"What? Is this true?" Jankhana screamed.

"We're pregnant! And it's a girl!" I burst out, no longer able to contain my excitement.

The room erupted into tears and laughter, squeals of joy and congratulations, and joking reprimands for not telling them all sooner —it was totally out of control and I loved every second of it. I basked in the glory of this moment. Samir and I had worked so hard to bring this life into being. For once, I felt like I was exactly where I was meant to be.

*   *   *

The rest of my pregnancy was a textbook case, as Dr. Coffman liked to call it. Once I reached eleven weeks, I "graduated" from the fertility clinic and was able to see my regular OB-GYN. From then on each scan and test moving forward were considered normal. I walked around in complete peace and awe for nine months and continued to thank God every chance I got. Though I knew I wouldn't fully exhale until I was at term and holding my healthy baby in my arms.

Thankfully, Sianna Julie Patel was born healthy at 7 pounds, 20.5 inches, on a beautiful Thursday afternoon.

Often, as I watched baby Sianna sleep, my heart weighed heavy with so many emotions. It was hard to comprehend how much I loved this tiny life, this precious girl, more than anything else in this world. Would she know how much I fought for her? Would she know the sleepless nights, the tears that were shed? That we never gave up hope?

Of course, she will know. And so will her little sister, Kaia, who came into the world five years later. My daughters have been the light of my life in the darkest days. This they will know.

*   *   *

Sianna means "a gift from God" in Hebrew. When we pray, I often tell Sianna the story of how much we prayed for her. She replies by saying, "Mama, I prayed to come to you too." I stare at her in awe and I know that faith, no matter what it looks like for each person, is what you need to help you find the life you are meant to lead.

EPILOGUE:
WHAT IS MEANT TO BE

I celebrated my first Mother's Day on May 10, 2015, more than two years after Samir and I began our fertility journey. To be sure, it was a happy and joyous occasion that we had worked very hard to arrive at. I wanted to savor the moment—the ups and downs, the struggle, the desperation to do whatever it takes, the willingness to go to any extreme—now that we had finally made the family we so desired.

I took a virtual stroll through my pictures and Facebook page, scrolling past so many memories: dancing in the crowd at the Grammys, our wedding day, seeing Depeche Mode live at Shoreline Amphitheater, wine-tasting in Napa Valley with Manish and Jana, Shaila's baby shower at the Art Institute of Chicago, Thanksgiving at Sudhir and Sonia's after our miscarriage, and the list goes on.

Those memories conjured up so many feelings. Good times and lots of laughter, but also sadness and heartache that were sometimes masked by putting up a brave front while we were with friends and family. I stopped when I got to a photo of me and Jankhana at NIU Sushi. That was the day I told her I was pregnant with my first pregnancy. It was very early on in the pregnancy and I had been advised not to tell others about it yet. But I was so giddy and excited. How could I have lunch with one of my best friends in the world and not tell her?

A pang of nostalgia thumped in my chest as I looked at the photo. I remembered how happy Jankhana had been when she heard the news. We both hugged and giggled like we were teenagers again and snapped a quick photo of the two of us before we left the restaurant. I had no idea then of the rough waters ahead. That the baby's chromosomal defect would prevent me from carrying him to term. That we would lose our little Peanut in the end.

The Facebook post was dated October 9, 2013. At the time, that date had no special significance for me. Looking at it again, though, it was as if I was seeing its importance for the first time. Sianna came into this world a healthy baby girl on October 9, 2014. She was born exactly one year to the day after that picture with Jankhana had been taken. And, in fact, I gave birth to her only one block away from the restaurant. If Facebook had a time stamp, I wonder if it would say 3:15 p.m., when Sianna entered this world. Not unlikely. Life works in mysteriously pleasant ways. What is meant to be is what will be.

*   *   *

When a woman goes through infertility challenges and finds herself traversing up a steep and winding road to motherhood, the entire process changes her to the core. The anxiety that comes along with years of trying, including fertility treatments, medications, the fear of the unknown, the conversations that are never had, and sometimes losing a baby, isn't something that just disappears one day. It is something that stays with you forever. I know this all too well. But we decided to choose hope over despair and never gave up, as much as we wanted to in those most challenging moments. The dream I had of my little girl didn't fail me.

Even when the future looks dark, look for signs. They are often the light that will help you to see what will be. I share our story out of a desire to bring optimism and courage to all the women around the world who struggle daily to get pregnant and carry their babies to term. If even just one woman takes a tiny bit of encouragement away from this journey, and it helps her keep her faith, my story is complete.

ACKNOWLEDGMENTS

The following acknowledgments come from the bottom of my heart and are in no particular order.

*   *   *

To those who have shared in our joy, pain, smiles, and tears, who have witnessed our daughters' births, who have lended a hand when we needed them, and who let me document their role in this book, thank you for coming on this journey with us. I hope as you read this, you will smile and know the impact you have had on our life. And I hope years down the line Sianna and Kaia will be the ones reading this, and they too will smile and know the impact our little tribe had on our family.

To Samir, we chose courage over fear, dedication over helplessness, faith over mistrust, and never stopped believing—for this I will always be grateful.

To my daughters, Sianna and Kaia, I am humbled to be your mom. You will always be my first and last thought, my greatest teachers, my smile, my joy, my sunshine, and my rocks. I would be nothing without you. I love you to infinity and beyond.

To Mom and Dad, thank you for loving me and supporting me unconditionally every single day.

To my Mother-in-law and Father-in-law, thank you for your love and support throughout this journey.

To Smita and Vikas, thank you for thinking of our baby's beautiful name.

To Jalpa, you will always be the wind beneath my wings. Your super powers as an author provided invaluable feedback on an early version of the book.

To Hetal and Jigish, we may be far in distance but you are in our thoughts every day.

To Megha, Sonya, Raj, and Arjun, we are so happy we were able to add to the Squad.

To my family and friends, the ones who have been there through the thick and thin of everyday life, thank you for always lifting me up and never ever letting me fall. You have carried me through some of my lowest days, and for that I will always be grateful.

To Taj, Nikiel, and Jaelan, you were the first who taught me how to love a tiny human with my whole being. When I met you, life gave me a new purpose. Thank you.

To my cousin Tina, at seventeen our worlds became one. Thank you for becoming my second "big sis" since then.

To my friend Reshma Saujani, as kids we were dreamers, today we are living them. Thank you for walking through this life with me.

To Roland, thanks for the pregnancy advice whenever we needed it. Your knowledge of your profession is immeasurable.

To Gunjan, Alpa, Rupal, and Rupa, we are as different as can be but somehow came from the same pod. Thanks to you I've lived two lives in this lifetime. You all have taught me more than you will ever know. Thank you for being my sisters.

To my friend Jankhana, I never imagined I would meet someone to walk hand in hand, side by side, in sync with me through every twist and turn of this life. Thank you.

To Shaila, we grew up oceans apart, one dinner brought us together. My life would not be the same without you. Thank you.

To Katie Salisbury, without you this memoir would not be possible. You are smart, kind, patient, knowledgeable, creative, and truly the best. You have guided me so patiently the last couple of years, I will always and forever be grateful to you.

To my doctor, thank you for believing in me.

ABOUT THE AUTHOR

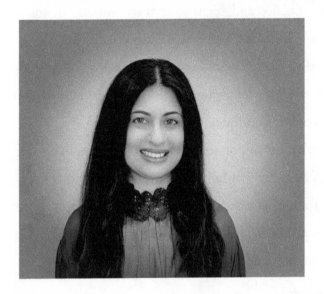

Julie Pandya Patel was born in India and immigrated to America with her family when she was just one year old. She grew up in the Northwest suburbs of Chicago and was an avid reader from a young age. Her work ethic and drive to help others was evident from a young age. As the daughter of Indian immigrants, she watched her parents work hard and make something of themselves in America, even though they arrived with just a few dollars in their pockets. Their values and dedication stuck with her.

After college, she was recruited at a job fair by a financial institution and embarked on a successful career in the finance sector that spanned more than fifteen years. Then in 2008, she took a brief hiatus from finance and spent four years working in the nonprofit world, helping individuals with disabilities on a national level. In 2012, she returned to the financial sector, taking a position at a top firm in Chicago. Today she's following her lifelong passion for fashion and has a successful online boutique.

Julie's most important job to date has been becoming a mom. *What Will Be* is her first book, a heartfelt memoir that holds nothing back with the aim of offering hope and encouragement to others who are struggling with infertility. Julie lives with her husband, Samir Patel, and their daughters, Sianna and Kaia, in Chicago.

9 781087 954264